Daily Journal

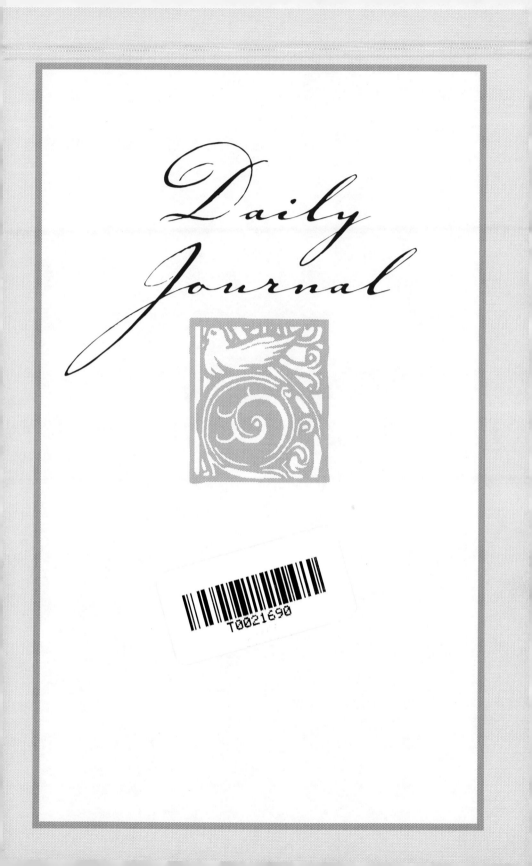

T0021690

THE GET WITH THE PROGRAM!

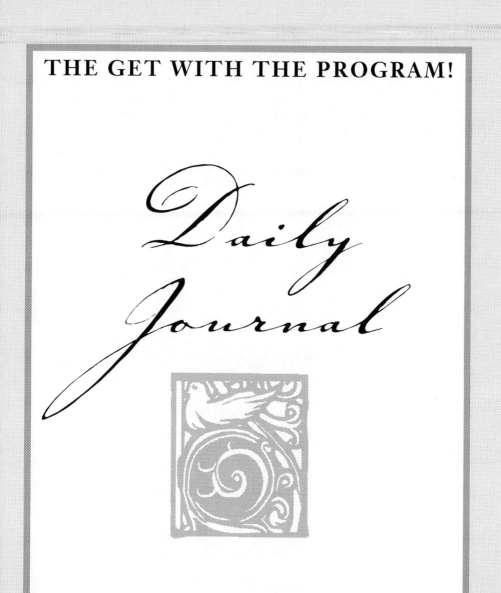

Daily Journal

BOB GREENE

SIMON & SCHUSTER

New York London Toronto Sydney

This publication contains the opinions and ideas of its author. It is intended to provide helpful and informative material on the subjects addressed in the publication. It is sold with the understanding that the author and publisher are not engaged in rendering medical, health, psychological, or any other kind of personal professional services in the book. If the reader requires personal medical, health, or other assistance or advice, a competent professional should be consulted.

The author and publisher specifically disclaim all responsibility for any liability, loss, or risk, personal or otherwise, that is incurred as a consequence, directly or indirectly, of the use and application of any of the contents of this book.

S

SIMON & SCHUSTER
Rockefeller Center
1230 Avenue of the Americas
New York, NY 10020

Copyright © 2002 by Bob Greene
All rights reserved, including the right of reproduction
in whole or in part in any form.

Simon & Schuster   and colophon are trademarks
of Simon & Schuster, Inc.

Make the Connection   and Get With the Program   are registered trademarks of Harpo, Inc.

For information regarding special discounts for bulk purchases,
please contact Simon & Schuster Special Sales:
1-800-456-6798 or business@simonandschuster.com

DESIGNED BY BONNI LEON   -BERMAN

Manufactured in the United States of America

1 3 5 7 9 10 8 6 4 2

ISBN 0-978-1-4516-5773-9

Introduction

Now that you've made the commitment to Get With the Program, you'll find that your new Daily Journal can be an invaluable tool, helping you to organize your nutrition and exercise goals for up to twelve weeks. Your journal will also help you take control of your emotional eating by giving you a safe and private place to express your feelings at those critical moments when you're most tempted by unwanted eating behavior.

Congratulations on making the commitment to Get With the Program. With the purchase of this daily journal, you're entitled to a free trial membership to the Get With the Program website. Simply log on to Getwiththeprogram.org and start enjoying all the unique benefits that your membership provides.

Before you begin your journal entries, it's a good idea to record some health information. In the spaces provided, fill in your starting weight, blood pressure, total cholesterol, LDL cholesterol, HDL cholesterol, blood sugar (glucose), and any body circumference measurements you wish to record.

Each day record the date, the week, and the current phase of your program. Then simply record all of the information that applies to your program phase and whether you met each goal of that phase.

The writing space is provided for you to record information about your eating patterns and/or habits. You should write about any eating episodes that are negative *or* positive. This will help you uncover the feelings and eating patterns that are related to your emotional eating. As you become more conscious of your eating triggers and patterns, you'll be better prepared for the "critical moment" that occurs right before you give in to emotional eating.

As I said in *Get With the Program!*, the best time to write in your journal is the moment *before* you begin emotional eating. Write down everything you can about each episode, including what you're feeling. Instead of eating, ask yourself the tough question about what's eating *you*. You might also want to write down other things you can do that will get you past this moment of temptation. The simple habit of going to your journal and writing before eating will eliminate much of your emotional eating. Remember: the best part about using your journal to help you eliminate your emotional eating is that you will more easily confront what needs to change in your life, and make improvements that you may not have thought of or have previously been unwilling to make.

Above all, enjoy your unique life journey.

GENERAL HEALTH INFORMATION

Consult your physician before you Get With the Program. Record the information you receive below:

Weight_____
Blood Pressure _____Systolic _____Diastolic

Total Cholesterol_____
LDL_____   HDL_____

Blood Glucose_____

Initial Measurements *(optional)*
Chest_____ Waist_____ Hips_____

Goals

GOALS FOR PHASE ONE

Explore your beliefs, attitudes, and behaviors that relate to yourself and the process of change.

Learn all about the process of how you gain and lose weight.

Drink a minimum of 6 eight-ounce glasses of water each day.

Start moving more and performing one set of fifteen repetitions of the basic functional fitness exercises three times per week.

Prepare yourself for a lifetime of being healthy and fit.

Recommended time at Phase One: one to three weeks.

GOALS FOR PHASE TWO

Drink a minimum of 7 eight-ounce glasses of water each day.

Increase your functional exercise routine to one set of fifteen, four times per week.

Perform aerobic exercise for a minimum of fifty minutes per week.

Begin to limit, or eliminate, your consumption of alcohol.

If you want to progress, increase your aerobic exercise to seventy-five minutes per week as you prepare for Phase Three.

Maintain your exercise log.

Recommended time at Phase Two: one to three months.

GOALS FOR PHASE THREE

Begin to understand the causes of and limit or eliminate your emotional eating.

Drink a minimum of 8 eight-ounce glasses of water each day.

Increase your functional exercises to two sets of fifteen repetitions of each exercise, five times per week

Increase your aerobic exercise to a minimum of 100 minutes per week.

If you want to progress, increase your aerobic exercise to 125 minutes per week as you prepare for Phase Four.

Continue to limit or eliminate your consumption of alcohol.

Maintain your exercise log.

Recommended time at Phase Three: one to three months.

GOALS FOR PHASE FOUR

Drink a minimum of 9 eight-ounce glasses of water each day.

Increase your functional exercises to three sets of fifteen repetitions each, five times per week.

Increase your aerobic exercise to a minimum of 150 minutes per week. Continue to increase the number and intensity of your weekly aerobic minutes according to your goals.

Incorporate the Essential Eight strength training exercises into your weekly exercise routine, three times a week (one set to start, progressing to three sets, according to your goals).

Continue to limit or eliminate your consumption of alcohol.

Continue to limit or eliminate your emotional eating.

Fine-tune your eating by instituting the "Limit 24-7" nutritional guideline at least five times a week.

Maintain your exercise log.

Recommended time at Phase Four: the rest of your life!

Daily Journal

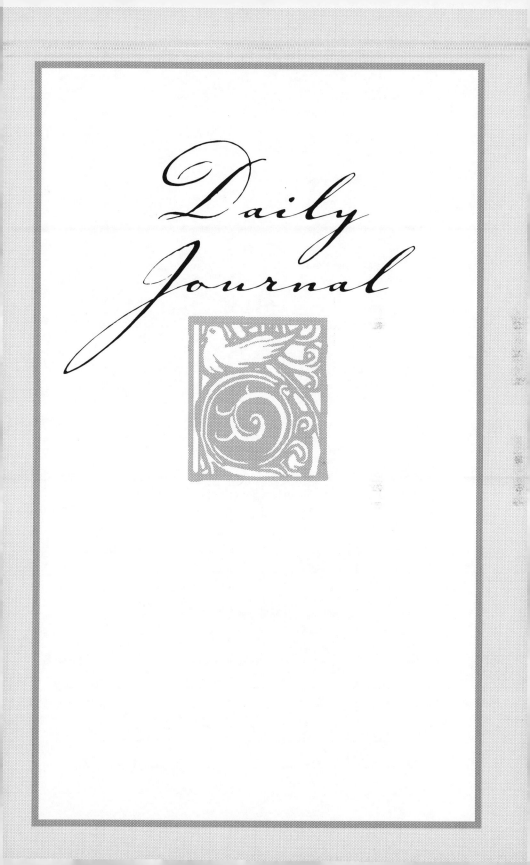

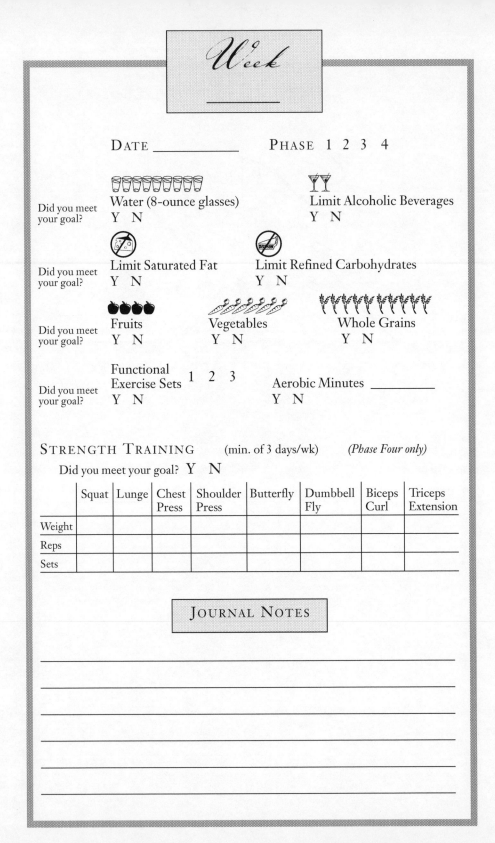

Week
_____

DATE _____   PHASE 1 2 3 4

Did you meet your goal?
Water (8-ounce glasses)
Y N

Limit Alcoholic Beverages
Y N

Did you meet your goal?
Limit Saturated Fat
Y N

Limit Refined Carbohydrates
Y N

Did you meet your goal?
Fruits
Y N

Vegetables
Y N

Whole Grains
Y N

Did you meet your goal?
Functional Exercise Sets   1   2   3
Y N

Aerobic Minutes _____
Y N

STRENGTH TRAINING   (min. of 3 days/wk)   *(Phase Four only)*

Did you meet your goal? Y N

	Squat	Lunge	Chest Press	Shoulder Press	Butterfly	Dumbbell Fly	Biceps Curl	Triceps Extension
Weight								
Reps								
Sets								

JOURNAL NOTES

_____

_____

_____

_____

_____

_____

> *The real challenge is to take a good, hard, honest look at yourself and summon up the courage to make permanent, positive changes in the way you think and behave.*

_____

_____

_____

_____

_____

_____

_____

_____

_____

_____

_____

_____

_____

_____

_____

_____

_____

_____

_____

_____

_____

_____

_____

_____

DATE _____   PHASE 1 2 3 4

Water (8-ounce glasses)

Did you meet
your goal?   Y N

Limit Alcoholic Beverages
Y N

Did you meet   Limit Saturated Fat   Limit Refined Carbohydrates
your goal?   Y N   Y N

Fruits   Vegetables   Whole Grains
Did you meet   Y N   Y N   Y N
your goal?

Functional
Exercise Sets   1 2 3
Did you meet   Aerobic Minutes _____
your goal?   Y N   Y N

STRENGTH TRAINING   (min. of 3 days/wk)   (Phase Four only)

Did you meet your goal? Y N

	Squat	Lunge	Chest Press	Shoulder Press	Butterfly	Dumbbell Fly	Biceps Curl	Triceps Extension
Weight								
Reps								
Sets								

JOURNAL NOTES

_____

_____

_____

_____

_____

_____

DATE _____   PHASE 1 2 3 4

Did you meet
your goal?   Water (8-ounce glasses)   Limit Alcoholic Beverages
                    Y N   Y N

Did you meet   Limit Saturated Fat   Limit Refined Carbohydrates
your goal?   Y N   Y N

Did you meet   Fruits   Vegetables   Whole Grains
your goal?   Y N   Y N   Y N

Did you meet   Functional
your goal?   Exercise Sets   1 2 3   Aerobic Minutes _____
                    Y N   Y N

STRENGTH TRAINING   (min. of 3 days/wk)   *(Phase Four only)*
    Did you meet your goal? Y N

	Squat	Lunge	Chest Press	Shoulder Press	Butterfly	Dumbbell Fly	Biceps Curl	Triceps Extension
Weight								
Reps								
Sets								

JOURNAL NOTES

_____

_____

_____

_____

_____

_____

DATE _____   PHASE 1 2 3 4

Did you meet your goal?   Water (8-ounce glasses)   Limit Alcoholic Beverages
                          Y N   Y N

Did you meet your goal?   Limit Saturated Fat   Limit Refined Carbohydrates
                          Y N   Y N

Did you meet your goal?   Fruits   Vegetables   Whole Grains
                          Y N   Y N   Y N

Did you meet your goal?   Functional   1 2 3
                          Exercise Sets   Aerobic Minutes _____
                          Y N   Y N

STRENGTH TRAINING   (min. of 3 days/wk)   *(Phase Four only)*

Did you meet your goal? Y N

	Squat	Lunge	Chest Press	Shoulder Press	Butterfly	Dumbbell Fly	Biceps Curl	Triceps Extension
Weight								
Reps								
Sets								

JOURNAL NOTES

_____

_____

_____

_____

_____

_____

DATE _____   PHASE 1 2 3 4

Did you meet
your goal?
Water (8-ounce glasses)
Y N

Limit Alcoholic Beverages
Y N

Did you meet
your goal?
Limit Saturated Fat
Y N

Limit Refined Carbohydrates
Y N

Did you meet
your goal?
Fruits
Y N

Vegetables
Y N

Whole Grains
Y N

Did you meet
your goal?
Functional
Exercise Sets   1   2   3
Y N

Aerobic Minutes _____
Y N

STRENGTH TRAINING   (min. of 3 days/wk)   *(Phase Four only)*

Did you meet your goal? Y N

	Squat	Lunge	Chest Press	Shoulder Press	Butterfly	Dumbbell Fly	Biceps Curl	Triceps Extension
Weight								
Reps								
Sets								

JOURNAL NOTES

_____

_____

_____

_____

_____

_____

DATE _____   PHASE 1 2 3 4

Water (8-ounce glasses)   Limit Alcoholic Beverages

Did you meet
your goal?   Y N   Y N

Limit Saturated Fat   Limit Refined Carbohydrates

Did you meet
your goal?   Y N   Y N

Fruits   Vegetables   Whole Grains

Did you meet
your goal?   Y N   Y N   Y N

Functional
Exercise Sets   1   2   3

Did you meet   Aerobic Minutes _____
your goal?   Y N   Y N

STRENGTH TRAINING   (min. of 3 days/wk)   *(Phase Four only)*

Did you meet your goal? Y N

	Squat	Lunge	Chest Press	Shoulder Press	Butterfly	Dumbbell Fly	Biceps Curl	Triceps Extension
Weight								
Reps								
Sets								

JOURNAL NOTES

_____

_____

_____

_____

_____

_____

DATE _____   PHASE 1 2 3 4

Did you meet
your goal?

Water (8-ounce glasses)   Limit Alcoholic Beverages
Y N   Y N

Did you meet
your goal?

Limit Saturated Fat   Limit Refined Carbohydrates
Y N   Y N

Did you meet
your goal?

Fruits   Vegetables   Whole Grains
Y N   Y N   Y N

Did you meet
your goal?

Functional
Exercise Sets 1 2 3   Aerobic Minutes _____
Y N   Y N

STRENGTH TRAINING   (min. of 3 days/wk)   *(Phase Four only)*

Did you meet your goal? Y N

	Squat	Lunge	Chest Press	Shoulder Press	Butterfly	Dumbbell Fly	Biceps Curl	Triceps Extension
Weight								
Reps								
Sets								

JOURNAL NOTES

_____

_____

_____

_____

_____

_____

> *Creating positive behavior in your life is what makes the difference between a successful fitness and weight-loss program and a failed one.*

_____

_____

_____

_____

_____

_____

_____

_____

_____

_____

_____

_____

_____

_____

_____

WEEKLY SUMMARY   *Body Weight*_____

	Water (8-ounce Glasses)	Functional Exercises	Aerobic Minutes	Number Alcoholic Beverages	Strength Training Sessions	"Limit 24-7" (All four)	Good Day or Not?
Monday							
Tuesday							
Wednesday							
Thursday							
Friday							
Saturday							
Sunday							

DATE _____   PHASE 1 2 3 4

Did you meet
your goal?

Water (8-ounce glasses)
Y N

Limit Alcoholic Beverages
Y N

Did you meet
your goal?

Limit Saturated Fat
Y N

Limit Refined Carbohydrates
Y N

Did you meet
your goal?

Fruits
Y N

Vegetables
Y N

Whole Grains
Y N

Did you meet
your goal?

Functional
Exercise Sets   1   2   3
Y N

Aerobic Minutes _____
Y N

STRENGTH TRAINING   (min. of 3 days/wk)   *(Phase Four only)*

Did you meet your goal? Y N

	Squat	Lunge	Chest Press	Shoulder Press	Butterfly	Dumbbell Fly	Biceps Curl	Triceps Extension
Weight								
Reps								
Sets								

JOURNAL NOTES

_____

_____

_____

_____

_____

_____

If you cut your calories without first increasing the amount of exercise you perform, your metabolism starts to shut down.

DATE _____   PHASE 1 2 3 4

Did you meet your goal?   Water (8-ounce glasses)   Limit Alcoholic Beverages
                           Y N   Y N

Did you meet your goal?   Limit Saturated Fat   Limit Refined Carbohydrates
                           Y N   Y N

Did you meet your goal?   Fruits   Vegetables   Whole Grains
                           Y N   Y N   Y N

Did you meet your goal?   Functional Exercise Sets 1 2 3   Aerobic Minutes _____
                           Y N   Y N

STRENGTH TRAINING   (min. of 3 days/wk)   *(Phase Four only)*

Did you meet your goal? Y N

	Squat	Lunge	Chest Press	Shoulder Press	Butterfly	Dumbbell Fly	Biceps Curl	Triceps Extension
Weight								
Reps								
Sets								

JOURNAL NOTES

_____

_____

_____

_____

_____

_____

DATE _____   PHASE   1 2 3 4

Did you meet
your goal?

Water (8-ounce glasses)
Y N

Limit Alcoholic Beverages
Y N

Did you meet
your goal?

Limit Saturated Fat
Y N

Limit Refined Carbohydrates
Y N

Did you meet
your goal?

Fruits
Y N

Vegetables
Y N

Whole Grains
Y N

Did you meet
your goal?

Functional
Exercise Sets   1   2   3
Y N

Aerobic Minutes _____
Y N

STRENGTH TRAINING   (min. of 3 days/wk)   *(Phase Four only)*

Did you meet your goal? Y N

	Squat	Lunge	Chest Press	Shoulder Press	Butterfly	Dumbbell Fly	Biceps Curl	Triceps Extension
Weight								
Reps								
Sets								

JOURNAL NOTES

_____

_____

_____

_____

_____

_____

DATE _____   PHASE 1 2 3 4

Water (8-ounce glasses)

Did you meet your goal?
Y N

Limit Alcoholic Beverages
Y N

Limit Saturated Fat

Did you meet your goal?
Y N

Limit Refined Carbohydrates
Y N

Fruits

Vegetables

Whole Grains

Did you meet your goal?
Y N

Y N

Y N

Functional Exercise Sets   1 2 3

Did you meet your goal?
Y N

Aerobic Minutes _____
Y N

STRENGTH TRAINING   (min. of 3 days/wk)   *(Phase Four only)*

Did you meet your goal? Y N

	Squat	Lunge	Chest Press	Shoulder Press	Butterfly	Dumbbell Fly	Biceps Curl	Triceps Extension
Weight								
Reps								
Sets								

JOURNAL NOTES

_____

_____

_____

_____

_____

_____

DATE _____   PHASE 1 2 3 4

Did you meet your goal?
Water (8-ounce glasses)
Y N

Limit Alcoholic Beverages
Y N

Did you meet your goal?
Limit Saturated Fat
Y N

Limit Refined Carbohydrates
Y N

Did you meet your goal?
Fruits
Y N

Vegetables
Y N

Whole Grains
Y N

Did you meet your goal?
Functional Exercise Sets 1 2 3
Y N

Aerobic Minutes _____
Y N

STRENGTH TRAINING   (min. of 3 days/wk)   *(Phase Four only)*

Did you meet your goal? Y N

	Squat	Lunge	Chest Press	Shoulder Press	Butterfly	Dumbbell Fly	Biceps Curl	Triceps Extension
Weight								
Reps								
Sets								

JOURNAL NOTES

_____

_____

_____

_____

_____

_____

DATE _____   PHASE 1 2 3 4

Did you meet
your goal?
Water (8-ounce glasses)   Limit Alcoholic Beverages
Y N   Y N

Did you meet
your goal?
Limit Saturated Fat   Limit Refined Carbohydrates
Y N   Y N

Did you meet
your goal?
Fruits   Vegetables   Whole Grains
Y N   Y N   Y N

Did you meet
your goal?
Functional
Exercise Sets 1 2 3
Y N   Aerobic Minutes _____
                              Y N

STRENGTH TRAINING   (min. of 3 days/wk)   *(Phase Four only)*

Did you meet your goal? Y N

	Squat	Lunge	Chest Press	Shoulder Press	Butterfly	Dumbbell Fly	Biceps Curl	Triceps Extension
Weight								
Reps								
Sets								

JOURNAL NOTES

_____

_____

_____

_____

_____

_____

DATE _____   PHASE   1   2   3   4

Water (8-ounce glasses)   Limit Alcoholic Beverages

Did you meet
your goal?
Y   N   Y   N

Limit Saturated Fat   Limit Refined Carbohydrates

Did you meet
your goal?
Y   N   Y   N

Fruits   Vegetables   Whole Grains

Did you meet
your goal?
Y   N   Y   N   Y   N

Functional
Exercise Sets   1   2   3
Did you meet
your goal?   Aerobic Minutes _____
Y   N   Y   N

STRENGTH TRAINING   (min. of 3 days/wk)   *(Phase Four only)*

Did you meet your goal? Y   N

	Squat	Lunge	Chest Press	Shoulder Press	Butterfly	Dumbbell Fly	Biceps Curl	Triceps Extension
Weight								
Reps								
Sets								

JOURNAL NOTES

_____

_____

_____

_____

_____

_____

> *It takes patience, persistence, and a positive attitude to lose weight the right way.*

_____
_____
_____
_____
_____
_____
_____
_____
_____
_____
_____
_____
_____
_____
_____
_____

WEEKLY SUMMARY   *Body Weight_____*

	Water (8-ounce Glasses)	Functional Exercises	Aerobic Minutes	Number Alcoholic Beverages	Strength Training Sessions	"Limit 24-7" (All four)	Good Day or Not?
Monday							
Tuesday							
Wednesday							
Thursday							
Friday							
Saturday							
Sunday							

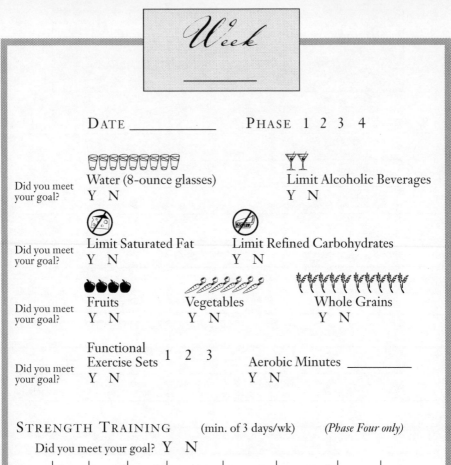

Week
_____

DATE _____   PHASE 1 2 3 4

Did you meet   Water (8-ounce glasses)   Limit Alcoholic Beverages
your goal?   Y N   Y N

Did you meet   Limit Saturated Fat   Limit Refined Carbohydrates
your goal?   Y N   Y N

Did you meet   Fruits   Vegetables   Whole Grains
your goal?   Y N   Y N   Y N

                Functional
Did you meet   Exercise Sets 1 2 3
your goal?   Y N   Aerobic Minutes _____
                                          Y N

STRENGTH TRAINING   (min. of 3 days/wk)   _(Phase Four only)_

Did you meet your goal? Y N

	Squat	Lunge	Chest Press	Shoulder Press	Butterfly	Dumbbell Fly	Biceps Curl	Triceps Extension
Weight								
Reps								
Sets								

JOURNAL NOTES

_____
_____
_____
_____
_____
_____

*Getting With the Program is about
self-discipline, self-control, and personal
commitment. Most of all, it's about feeling good
about yourself and taking good care of yourself.*

_____
_____
_____
_____
_____
_____
_____
_____
_____
_____
_____
_____
_____
_____
_____
_____
_____
_____
_____
_____
_____
_____
_____
_____
_____
_____

DATE _____   PHASE 1 2 3 4

Did you meet
your goal?
Water (8-ounce glasses)
Y N

Limit Alcoholic Beverages
Y N

Did you meet
your goal?
Limit Saturated Fat
Y N

Limit Refined Carbohydrates
Y N

Did you meet
your goal?
Fruits
Y N

Vegetables
Y N

Whole Grains
Y N

Did you meet
your goal?
Functional
Exercise Sets 1 2 3
Y N

Aerobic Minutes _____
Y N

STRENGTH TRAINING   (min. of 3 days/wk)   *(Phase Four only)*

Did you meet your goal? Y N

	Squat	Lunge	Chest Press	Shoulder Press	Butterfly	Dumbbell Fly	Biceps Curl	Triceps Extension
Weight								
Reps								
Sets								

JOURNAL NOTES

_____

_____

_____

_____

_____

_____

DATE _____ PHASE 1 2 3 4

Water (8-ounce glasses)

Did you meet
your goal?
Y N

Limit Alcoholic Beverages
Y N

Limit Saturated Fat

Did you meet
your goal?
Y N

Limit Refined Carbohydrates
Y N

Fruits

Vegetables

Whole Grains

Did you meet
your goal?
Y N

Y N

Y N

Did you meet
your goal?

Functional
Exercise Sets   1   2   3
Y N

Aerobic Minutes _____
Y N

STRENGTH TRAINING   (min. of 3 days/wk)   *(Phase Four only)*

Did you meet your goal? Y N

	Squat	Lunge	Chest Press	Shoulder Press	Butterfly	Dumbbell Fly	Biceps Curl	Triceps Extension
Weight								
Reps								
Sets								

JOURNAL NOTES

_____

_____

_____

_____

_____

_____

DATE _____   PHASE 1 2 3 4

Did you meet
your goal?
Water (8-ounce glasses)
Y N

Limit Alcoholic Beverages
Y N

Did you meet
your goal?
Limit Saturated Fat
Y N

Limit Refined Carbohydrates
Y N

Did you meet
your goal?
Fruits
Y N

Vegetables
Y N

Whole Grains
Y N

Did you meet
your goal?
Functional
Exercise Sets   1   2   3
Y N

Aerobic Minutes _____
Y N

STRENGTH TRAINING   (min. of 3 days/wk)   *(Phase Four only)*

Did you meet your goal? Y N

	Squat	Lunge	Chest Press	Shoulder Press	Butterfly	Dumbbell Fly	Biceps Curl	Triceps Extension
Weight								
Reps								
Sets								

JOURNAL NOTES

_____

_____

_____

_____

_____

_____

DATE _____ PHASE 1 2 3 4

Did you meet your goal?
Water (8-ounce glasses)
Y N

Limit Alcoholic Beverages
Y N

Did you meet your goal?
Limit Saturated Fat
Y N

Limit Refined Carbohydrates
Y N

Did you meet your goal?
Fruits
Y N

Vegetables
Y N

Whole Grains
Y N

Did you meet your goal?
Functional Exercise Sets 1 2 3
Y N

Aerobic Minutes _____
Y N

STRENGTH TRAINING (min. of 3 days/wk) *(Phase Four only)*

Did you meet your goal? Y N

	Squat	Lunge	Chest Press	Shoulder Press	Butterfly	Dumbbell Fly	Biceps Curl	Triceps Extension
Weight								
Reps								
Sets								

JOURNAL NOTES

_____

_____

_____

_____

_____

_____

DATE _____   PHASE 1 2 3 4

Water (8-ounce glasses)   Limit Alcoholic Beverages

Did you meet
your goal?   Y N   Y N

Limit Saturated Fat   Limit Refined Carbohydrates

Did you meet
your goal?   Y N   Y N

Fruits   Vegetables   Whole Grains

Did you meet
your goal?   Y N   Y N   Y N

Functional   1 2 3
Exercise Sets
Did you meet   Aerobic Minutes _____
your goal?   Y N   Y N

STRENGTH TRAINING   (min. of 3 days/wk)   *(Phase Four only)*

Did you meet your goal? Y N

	Squat	Lunge	Chest Press	Shoulder Press	Butterfly	Dumbbell Fly	Biceps Curl	Triceps Extension
Weight								
Reps								
Sets								

JOURNAL NOTES

_____

_____

_____

_____

_____

_____

DATE _____   PHASE   1   2   3   4

Did you meet
your goal?

Water (8-ounce glasses)   Limit Alcoholic Beverages
Y N   Y N

Did you meet
your goal?

Limit Saturated Fat   Limit Refined Carbohydrates
Y N   Y N

Did you meet
your goal?

Fruits   Vegetables   Whole Grains
Y N   Y N   Y N

Did you meet
your goal?

Functional
Exercise Sets   1   2   3   Aerobic Minutes _____
Y N   Y N

STRENGTH TRAINING   (min. of 3 days/wk)   *(Phase Four only)*

Did you meet your goal? Y N

	Squat	Lunge	Chest Press	Shoulder Press	Butterfly	Dumbbell Fly	Biceps Curl	Triceps Extension
Weight								
Reps								
Sets								

JOURNAL NOTES

_____

_____

_____

_____

_____

_____

> *The way you think will ultimately dictate your long-term success or failure.*

_____

_____

_____

_____

_____

_____

_____

_____

_____

_____

_____

_____

_____

_____

_____

_____

WEEKLY SUMMARY   *Body Weight*_____

	Water (8-ounce Glasses)	Functional Exercises	Aerobic Minutes	Number Alcoholic Beverages	Strength Training Sessions	"Limit 24-7" (All four)	Good Day or Not?
Monday							
Tuesday							
Wednesday							
Thursday							
Friday							
Saturday							
Sunday							

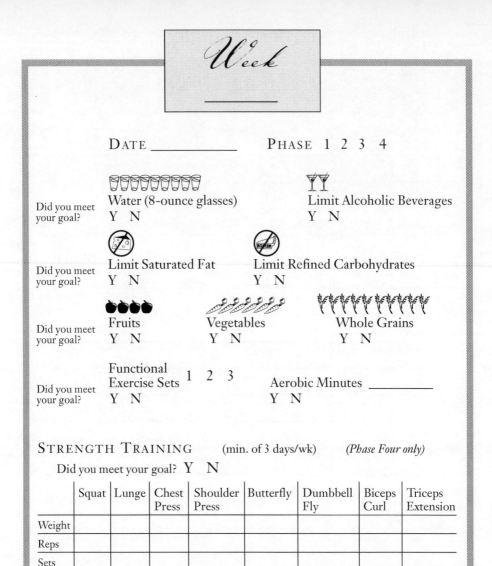

Week

DATE _____   PHASE 1 2 3 4

Water (8-ounce glasses)   Limit Alcoholic Beverages
Did you meet
your goal?   Y N   Y N

Limit Saturated Fat   Limit Refined Carbohydrates
Did you meet
your goal?   Y N   Y N

Fruits   Vegetables   Whole Grains
Did you meet
your goal?   Y N   Y N   Y N

Functional
Exercise Sets 1 2 3
Did you meet   Aerobic Minutes _____
your goal?   Y N   Y N

STRENGTH TRAINING   (min. of 3 days/wk)   *(Phase Four only)*

Did you meet your goal? Y N

	Squat	Lunge	Chest Press	Shoulder Press	Butterfly	Dumbbell Fly	Biceps Curl	Triceps Extension
Weight								
Reps								
Sets								

JOURNAL NOTES

_____
_____
_____
_____
_____
_____

*Taking responsibility means looking to yourself
to create your own life.*

DATE _____   PHASE 1 2 3 4

Did you meet   Water (8-ounce glasses)   Limit Alcoholic Beverages
your goal?   Y N   Y N

Did you meet   Limit Saturated Fat   Limit Refined Carbohydrates
your goal?   Y N   Y N

Did you meet   Fruits   Vegetables   Whole Grains
your goal?   Y N   Y N   Y N

                     Functional
Did you meet   Exercise Sets 1 2 3
your goal?   Y N   Aerobic Minutes _____
                                                    Y N

STRENGTH TRAINING   (min. of 3 days/wk)   *(Phase Four only)*

Did you meet your goal? Y N

	Squat	Lunge	Chest Press	Shoulder Press	Butterfly	Dumbbell Fly	Biceps Curl	Triceps Extension
Weight								
Reps								
Sets								

JOURNAL NOTES

_____

_____

_____

_____

_____

_____

DATE _____   PHASE 1 2 3 4

Did you meet
your goal?
Water (8-ounce glasses)
Y N

Limit Alcoholic Beverages
Y N

Did you meet
your goal?
Limit Saturated Fat
Y N

Limit Refined Carbohydrates
Y N

Did you meet
your goal?
Fruits
Y N

Vegetables
Y N

Whole Grains
Y N

Did you meet
your goal?
Functional
Exercise Sets 1 2 3
Y N

Aerobic Minutes _____
Y N

STRENGTH TRAINING   (min. of 3 days/wk)   *(Phase Four only)*
Did you meet your goal? Y N

	Squat	Lunge	Chest Press	Shoulder Press	Butterfly	Dumbbell Fly	Biceps Curl	Triceps Extension
Weight								
Reps								
Sets								

JOURNAL NOTES

_____

_____

_____

_____

_____

_____

DATE _____   PHASE 1 2 3 4

Did you meet
your goal?
Water (8-ounce glasses)
Y N

Limit Alcoholic Beverages
Y N

Did you meet
your goal?
Limit Saturated Fat
Y N

Limit Refined Carbohydrates
Y N

Did you meet
your goal?
Fruits
Y N

Vegetables
Y N

Whole Grains
Y N

Did you meet
your goal?
Functional
Exercise Sets   1   2   3
Y N

Aerobic Minutes _____
Y N

STRENGTH TRAINING   (min. of 3 days/wk)   *(Phase Four only)*

Did you meet your goal? Y N

	Squat	Lunge	Chest Press	Shoulder Press	Butterfly	Dumbbell Fly	Biceps Curl	Triceps Extension
Weight								
Reps								
Sets								

JOURNAL NOTES

_____

_____

_____

_____

_____

_____

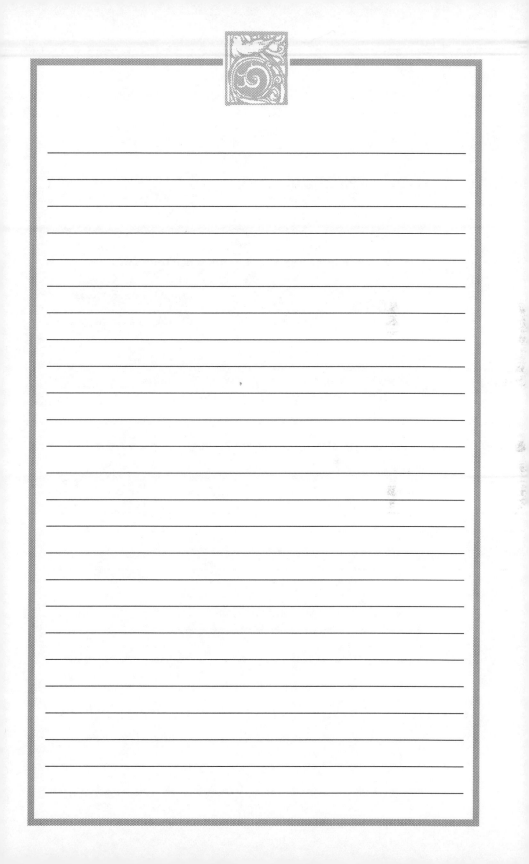

DATE _____   PHASE 1 2 3 4

Did you meet
your goal?
Water (8-ounce glasses)   Limit Alcoholic Beverages
Y N   Y N

Did you meet
your goal?
Limit Saturated Fat   Limit Refined Carbohydrates
Y N   Y N

Did you meet
your goal?
Fruits   Vegetables   Whole Grains
Y N   Y N   Y N

Did you meet
your goal?
Functional
Exercise Sets 1 2 3   . Aerobic Minutes _____
Y N   Y N

STRENGTH TRAINING   (min. of 3 days/wk)   *(Phase Four only)*

Did you meet your goal? Y N

	Squat	Lunge	Chest Press	Shoulder Press	Butterfly	Dumbbell Fly	Biceps Curl	Triceps Extension
Weight								
Reps								
Sets								

JOURNAL NOTES

_____

_____

_____

_____

_____

_____

DATE _____   PHASE 1 2 3 4

Did you meet your goal?
Water (8-ounce glasses)
Y N

Limit Alcoholic Beverages
Y N

Did you meet your goal?
Limit Saturated Fat
Y N

Limit Refined Carbohydrates
Y N

Did you meet your goal?
Fruits
Y N

Vegetables
Y N

Whole Grains
Y N

Did you meet your goal?
Functional Exercise Sets 1 2 3
Y N

Aerobic Minutes _____
Y N

STRENGTH TRAINING   (min. of 3 days/wk)   *(Phase Four only)*

Did you meet your goal? Y N

	Squat	Lunge	Chest Press	Shoulder Press	Butterfly	Dumbbell Fly	Biceps Curl	Triceps Extension
Weight								
Reps								
Sets								

JOURNAL NOTES

_____

_____

_____

_____

_____

_____

DATE _____   PHASE 1 2 3 4

Did you meet
your goal?
Water (8-ounce glasses)
Y N

Limit Alcoholic Beverages
Y N

Did you meet
your goal?
Limit Saturated Fat
Y N

Limit Refined Carbohydrates
Y N

Did you meet
your goal?
Fruits
Y N

Vegetables
Y N

Whole Grains
Y N

Did you meet
your goal?
Functional
Exercise Sets 1 2 3
Y N

Aerobic Minutes _____
Y N

STRENGTH TRAINING   (min. of 3 days/wk)   *(Phase Four only)*

Did you meet your goal? Y N

	Squat	Lunge	Chest Press	Shoulder Press	Butterfly	Dumbbell Fly	Biceps Curl	Triceps Extension
Weight								
Reps								
Sets								

JOURNAL NOTES

_____

_____

_____

_____

_____

_____

_____

_____

_____

_____

_____

_____

_____

_____

_____

_____

_____

_____

_____

_____

_____

_____

WEEKLY SUMMARY   *Body Weight*_____

	Water (8-ounce Glasses)	Functional Exercises	Aerobic Minutes	Number Alcoholic Beverages	Strength Training Sessions	"Limit 24-7" (All four)	Good Day or Not?
Monday							
Tuesday							
Wednesday							
Thursday							
Friday							
Saturday							
Sunday							

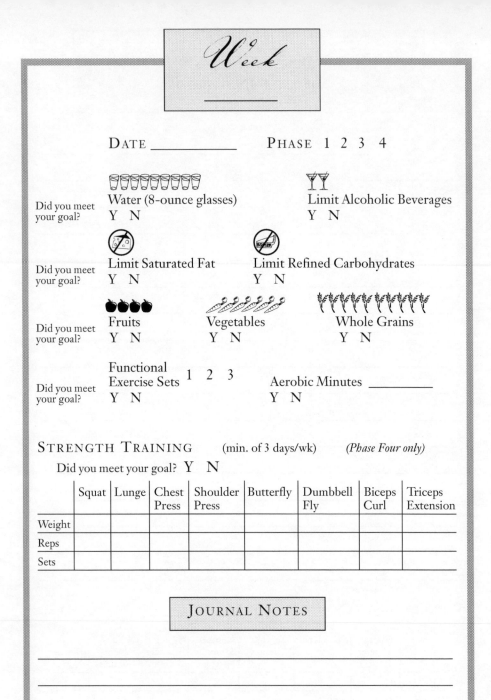

$\mathscr{W}\!eek$

_____

DATE _____   PHASE 1 2 3 4

Did you meet
your goal?
Water (8-ounce glasses)
Y N

Limit Alcoholic Beverages
Y N

Did you meet
your goal?
Limit Saturated Fat
Y N

Limit Refined Carbohydrates
Y N

Did you meet
your goal?
Fruits
Y N

Vegetables
Y N

Whole Grains
Y N

Did you meet
your goal?
Functional
Exercise Sets 1 2 3
Y N

Aerobic Minutes _____
Y N

STRENGTH TRAINING   (min. of 3 days/wk)   *(Phase Four only)*

Did you meet your goal? Y N

	Squat	Lunge	Chest Press	Shoulder Press	Butterfly	Dumbbell Fly	Biceps Curl	Triceps Extension
Weight								
Reps								
Sets								

JOURNAL NOTES

_____

_____

_____

_____

_____

_____

*Be patient. If you can find or create things to
be happy about today, you'll be much more likely
to take care of yourself tomorrow.*

_____
_____
_____
_____
_____
_____
_____
_____
_____
_____
_____
_____
_____
_____
_____
_____
_____
_____
_____
_____
_____
_____
_____
_____

DATE _____   PHASE 1 2 3 4

Did you meet your goal?
Water (8-ounce glasses)
Y N

Limit Alcoholic Beverages
Y N

Did you meet your goal?
Limit Saturated Fat
Y N

Limit Refined Carbohydrates
Y N

Did you meet your goal?
Fruits
Y N

Vegetables
Y N

Whole Grains
Y N

Did you meet your goal?
Functional Exercise Sets   1   2   3
Y N

Aerobic Minutes _____
Y N

STRENGTH TRAINING   (min. of 3 days/wk)   *(Phase Four only)*

Did you meet your goal? Y N

	Squat	Lunge	Chest Press	Shoulder Press	Butterfly	Dumbbell Fly	Biceps Curl	Triceps Extension
Weight								
Reps								
Sets								

JOURNAL NOTES

_____

_____

_____

_____

_____

_____

DATE _____ PHASE 1 2 3 4

Did you meet
your goal?
Water (8-ounce glasses)
Y N

Limit Alcoholic Beverages
Y N

Did you meet
your goal?
Limit Saturated Fat
Y N

Limit Refined Carbohydrates
Y N

Did you meet
your goal?
Fruits
Y N

Vegetables
Y N

Whole Grains
Y N

Did you meet
your goal?
Functional
Exercise Sets   1   2   3
Y N

Aerobic Minutes _____
Y N

STRENGTH TRAINING   (min. of 3 days/wk)   *(Phase Four only)*

Did you meet your goal? Y N

	Squat	Lunge	Chest Press	Shoulder Press	Butterfly	Dumbbell Fly	Biceps Curl	Triceps Extension
Weight								
Reps								
Sets								

JOURNAL NOTES

_____

_____

_____

_____

_____

_____

DATE _____   PHASE 1 2 3 4

Did you meet your goal?
Water (8-ounce glasses)
Y N

Limit Alcoholic Beverages
Y N

Did you meet your goal?
Limit Saturated Fat
Y N

Limit Refined Carbohydrates
Y N

Did you meet your goal?
Fruits
Y N

Vegetables
Y N

Whole Grains
Y N

Did you meet your goal?
Functional Exercise Sets 1 2 3
Y N

Aerobic Minutes _____
Y N

STRENGTH TRAINING   (min. of 3 days/wk)   *(Phase Four only)*

Did you meet your goal? Y N

	Squat	Lunge	Chest Press	Shoulder Press	Butterfly	Dumbbell Fly	Biceps Curl	Triceps Extension
Weight								
Reps								
Sets								

JOURNAL NOTES

_____

_____

_____

_____

_____

_____

DATE _____ PHASE 1 2 3 4

Did you meet your goal? Water (8-ounce glasses)
Y N

Limit Alcoholic Beverages
Y N

Did you meet your goal? Limit Saturated Fat
Y N

Limit Refined Carbohydrates
Y N

Did you meet your goal? Fruits
Y N

Vegetables
Y N

Whole Grains
Y N

Did you meet your goal? Functional Exercise Sets 1 2 3
Y N

Aerobic Minutes _____
Y N

STRENGTH TRAINING   (min. of 3 days/wk)   (Phase Four only)

Did you meet your goal? Y N

	Squat	Lunge	Chest Press	Shoulder Press	Butterfly	Dumbbell Fly	Biceps Curl	Triceps Extension
Weight								
Reps								
Sets								

JOURNAL NOTES

_____

_____

_____

_____

_____

_____

DATE _____   PHASE 1 2 3 4

Did you meet
your goal?

Water (8-ounce glasses)
Y N

Limit Alcoholic Beverages
Y N

Did you meet
your goal?

Limit Saturated Fat
Y N

Limit Refined Carbohydrates
Y N

Did you meet
your goal?

Fruits
Y N

Vegetables
Y N

Whole Grains
Y N

Did you meet
your goal?

Functional
Exercise Sets   1   2   3
Y N

Aerobic Minutes _____
Y N

STRENGTH TRAINING   (min. of 3 days/wk)   *(Phase Four only)*

Did you meet your goal? Y N

	Squat	Lunge	Chest Press	Shoulder Press	Butterfly	Dumbbell Fly	Biceps Curl	Triceps Extension
Weight								
Reps								
Sets								

JOURNAL NOTES

_____

_____

_____

_____

_____

_____

DATE _____   PHASE 1 2 3 4

Did you meet
your goal?
Water (8-ounce glasses)   Limit Alcoholic Beverages
Y N   Y N

Did you meet
your goal?
Limit Saturated Fat   Limit Refined Carbohydrates
Y N   Y N

Did you meet
your goal?
Fruits   Vegetables   Whole Grains
Y N   Y N   Y N

Did you meet
your goal?
Functional
Exercise Sets   1   2   3
Y N   Aerobic Minutes _____
                                 Y N

STRENGTH TRAINING   (min. of 3 days/wk)   *(Phase Four only)*

Did you meet your goal? Y N

	Squat	Lunge	Chest Press	Shoulder Press	Butterfly	Dumbbell Fly	Biceps Curl	Triceps Extension
Weight								
Reps								
Sets								

JOURNAL NOTES

_____

_____

_____

_____

_____

_____

> *It's so important to establish a variety of goals in several aspects of your life.*

_____

_____

_____

_____

_____

_____

_____

_____

_____

_____

_____

_____

_____

_____

_____

_____

WEEKLY SUMMARY   *Body Weight*_____

	Water (8-ounce Glasses)	Functional Exercises	Aerobic Minutes	Number Alcoholic Beverages	Strength Training Sessions	"Limit 24-7" (All four)	Good Day or Not?
Monday							
Tuesday							
Wednesday							
Thursday							
Friday							
Saturday							
Sunday							

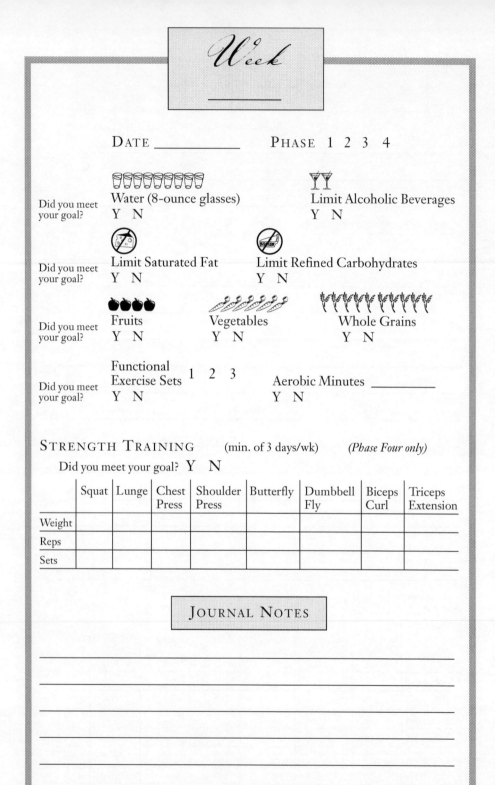

Week

DATE _____ PHASE 1 2 3 4

Did you meet your goal?   Water (8-ounce glasses)
Y N

Limit Alcoholic Beverages
Y N

Did you meet your goal?   Limit Saturated Fat
Y N

Limit Refined Carbohydrates
Y N

Did you meet your goal?   Fruits
Y N

Vegetables
Y N

Whole Grains
Y N

Did you meet your goal?   Functional Exercise Sets 1 2 3
Y N

Aerobic Minutes _____
Y N

STRENGTH TRAINING   (min. of 3 days/wk)   *(Phase Four only)*

Did you meet your goal? Y N

	Squat	Lunge	Chest Press	Shoulder Press	Butterfly	Dumbbell Fly	Biceps Curl	Triceps Extension
Weight								
Reps								
Sets								

JOURNAL NOTES

_____

_____

_____

_____

_____

_____

Dedication, commitment, and effort are needed to accomplish anything worthwhile.

DATE _____   PHASE 1 2 3 4

Did you meet
your goal?
Water (8-ounce glasses)
Y N

Limit Alcoholic Beverages
Y N

Did you meet
your goal?
Limit Saturated Fat
Y N

Limit Refined Carbohydrates
Y N

Did you meet
your goal?
Fruits
Y N

Vegetables
Y N

Whole Grains
Y N

Did you meet
your goal?
Functional
Exercise Sets   1   2   3
Y N

Aerobic Minutes _____
Y N

STRENGTH TRAINING   (min. of 3 days/wk)   *(Phase Four only)*

Did you meet your goal? Y N

	Squat	Lunge	Chest Press	Shoulder Press	Butterfly	Dumbbell Fly	Biceps Curl	Triceps Extension
Weight								
Reps								
Sets								

JOURNAL NOTES

_____

_____

_____

_____

_____

_____

DATE _____   PHASE   1   2   3   4

Did you meet your goal?   Water (8-ounce glasses)   Limit Alcoholic Beverages
                          Y   N   Y   N

Did you meet your goal?   Limit Saturated Fat   Limit Refined Carbohydrates
                          Y   N   Y   N

Did you meet your goal?   Fruits   Vegetables   Whole Grains
                          Y   N   Y   N   Y   N

Did you meet your goal?   Functional
                          Exercise Sets   1   2   3
                          Y   N   Aerobic Minutes _____
                                                      Y   N

STRENGTH TRAINING   (min. of 3 days/wk)   *(Phase Four only)*

Did you meet your goal? Y   N

	Squat	Lunge	Chest Press	Shoulder Press	Butterfly	Dumbbell Fly	Biceps Curl	Triceps Extension
Weight								
Reps								
Sets								

JOURNAL NOTES

_____

_____

_____

_____

_____

_____

DATE _____   PHASE 1 2 3 4

Did you meet
your goal?
Water (8-ounce glasses)
Y N

Limit Alcoholic Beverages
Y N

Did you meet
your goal?
Limit Saturated Fat
Y N

Limit Refined Carbohydrates
Y N

Did you meet
your goal?
Fruits
Y N

Vegetables
Y N

Whole Grains
Y N

Did you meet
your goal?
Functional
Exercise Sets 1 2 3
Y N

Aerobic Minutes _____
Y N

STRENGTH TRAINING   (min. of 3 days/wk)   *(Phase Four only)*

Did you meet your goal? Y N

	Squat	Lunge	Chest Press	Shoulder Press	Butterfly	Dumbbell Fly	Biceps Curl	Triceps Extension
Weight								
Reps								
Sets								

JOURNAL NOTES

_____

_____

_____

_____

_____

_____

DATE _____   PHASE 1 2 3 4

Water (8-ounce glasses)

Did you meet
your goal?   Y N

Limit Alcoholic Beverages
Y N

Did you meet
your goal?   Limit Saturated Fat   Limit Refined Carbohydrates
Y N   Y N

Did you meet
your goal?   Fruits   Vegetables   Whole Grains
Y N   Y N   Y N

Did you meet
your goal?   Functional
Exercise Sets   1   2   3
Y N   Aerobic Minutes _____
Y N

STRENGTH TRAINING   (min. of 3 days/wk)   *(Phase Four only)*

Did you meet your goal? Y N

	Squat	Lunge	Chest Press	Shoulder Press	Butterfly	Dumbbell Fly	Biceps Curl	Triceps Extension
Weight								
Reps								
Sets								

JOURNAL NOTES

_____

_____

_____

_____

_____

_____

DATE _____   PHASE   1 2 3   4

Did you meet your goal?   Water (8-ounce glasses)   Limit Alcoholic Beverages
                          Y   N   Y   N

Did you meet your goal?   Limit Saturated Fat   Limit Refined Carbohydrates
                          Y   N   Y   N

Did you meet your goal?   Fruits   Vegetables   Whole Grains
                          Y   N   Y   N   Y   N

Did you meet your goal?   Functional
                          Exercise Sets   1   2   3   Aerobic Minutes _____
                          Y   N   Y   N

STRENGTH TRAINING   (min. of 3 days/wk)   *(Phase Four only)*

Did you meet your goal?   Y   N

	Squat	Lunge	Chest Press	Shoulder Press	Butterfly	Dumbbell Fly	Biceps Curl	Triceps Extension
Weight								
Reps								
Sets								

JOURNAL NOTES

_____

_____

_____

_____

_____

_____

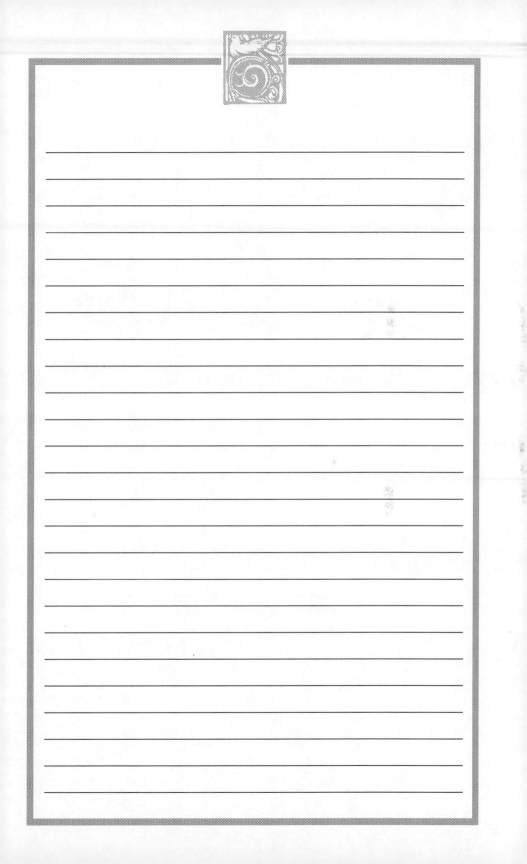

DATE _____   PHASE 1 2 3 4

Did you meet
your goal?
Water (8-ounce glasses)
Y N

Limit Alcoholic Beverages
Y N

Did you meet
your goal?
Limit Saturated Fat
Y N

Limit Refined Carbohydrates
Y N

Did you meet
your goal?
Fruits
Y N

Vegetables
Y N

Whole Grains
Y N

Did you meet
your goal?
Functional
Exercise Sets 1 2 3
Y N

Aerobic Minutes _____
Y N

STRENGTH TRAINING   (min. of 3 days/wk)   *(Phase Four only)*

Did you meet your goal? Y N

	Squat	Lunge	Chest Press	Shoulder Press	Butterfly	Dumbbell Fly	Biceps Curl	Triceps Extension
Weight								
Reps								
Sets								

JOURNAL NOTES

_____

_____

_____

_____

_____

_____

> *The easy way out will always look tempting when stacked up against hard work. But working hard and earning your results is exactly what increases your self-esteem.*

_____
_____
_____
_____
_____
_____
_____
_____
_____
_____
_____
_____
_____

WEEKLY SUMMARY   *Body Weight*_____

	Water (8-ounce Glasses)	Functional Exercises	Aerobic Minutes	Number Alcoholic Beverages	Strength Training Sessions	"Limit 24-7" (All four)	Good Day or Not?
Monday							
Tuesday							
Wednesday							
Thursday							
Friday							
Saturday							
Sunday							

$\mathcal{W}eek$

_____

DATE _____ PHASE 1 2 3 4

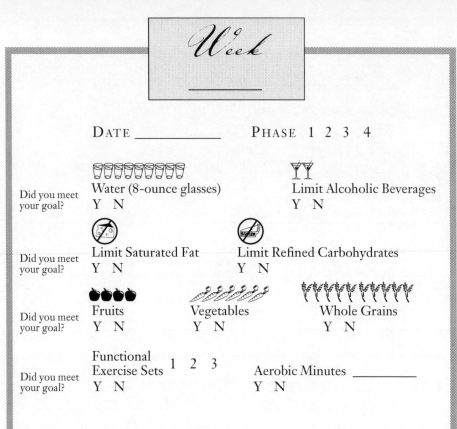

Did you meet your goal?
Water (8-ounce glasses)
Y N

Limit Alcoholic Beverages
Y N

Did you meet your goal?
Limit Saturated Fat
Y N

Limit Refined Carbohydrates
Y N

Did you meet your goal?
Fruits
Y N

Vegetables
Y N

Whole Grains
Y N

Did you meet your goal?
Functional Exercise Sets   1   2   3
Y N

Aerobic Minutes _____
Y N

STRENGTH TRAINING   (min. of 3 days/wk)   *(Phase Four only)*

Did you meet your goal? Y N

	Squat	Lunge	Chest Press	Shoulder Press	Butterfly	Dumbbell Fly	Biceps Curl	Triceps Extension
Weight								
Reps								
Sets								

JOURNAL NOTES

_____

_____

_____

_____

_____

_____

DATE _____   PHASE 1 2 3 4

Did you meet   Water (8-ounce glasses)   Limit Alcoholic Beverages
your goal?   Y N   Y N

Did you meet   Limit Saturated Fat   Limit Refined Carbohydrates
your goal?   Y N   Y N

Did you meet   Fruits   Vegetables   Whole Grains
your goal?   Y N   Y N   Y N

Did you meet   Functional
your goal?   Exercise Sets 1 2 3   Aerobic Minutes _____
                 Y N   Y N

STRENGTH TRAINING   (min. of 3 days/wk)   (Phase Four only)
Did you meet your goal? Y N

	Squat	Lunge	Chest Press	Shoulder Press	Butterfly	Dumbbell Fly	Biceps Curl	Triceps Extension
Weight								
Reps								
Sets								

JOURNAL NOTES

_____

_____

_____

_____

_____

_____

DATE _____   PHASE 1 2 3 4

Did you meet
your goal?

Water (8-ounce glasses)
Y N

Limit Alcoholic Beverages
Y N

Did you meet
your goal?

Limit Saturated Fat
Y N

Limit Refined Carbohydrates
Y N

Did you meet
your goal?

Fruits
Y N

Vegetables
Y N

Whole Grains
Y N

Did you meet
your goal?

Functional
Exercise Sets   1   2   3
Y N

Aerobic Minutes _____
Y N

STRENGTH TRAINING   (min. of 3 days/wk)   *(Phase Four only)*

Did you meet your goal? Y   N

	Squat	Lunge	Chest Press	Shoulder Press	Butterfly	Dumbbell Fly	Biceps Curl	Triceps Extension
Weight								
Reps								
Sets								

JOURNAL NOTES

_____

_____

_____

_____

_____

_____

DATE _____   PHASE 1 2 3 4

Did you meet
your goal?
Water (8-ounce glasses)
Y N

Limit Alcoholic Beverages
Y N

Did you meet
your goal?
Limit Saturated Fat
Y N

Limit Refined Carbohydrates
Y N

Did you meet
your goal?
Fruits
Y N

Vegetables
Y N

Whole Grains
Y N

Did you meet
your goal?
Functional
Exercise Sets 1 2 3
Y N

Aerobic Minutes _____
Y N

STRENGTH TRAINING   (min. of 3 days/wk)   *(Phase Four only)*

Did you meet your goal? Y N

	Squat	Lunge	Chest Press	Shoulder Press	Butterfly	Dumbbell Fly	Biceps Curl	Triceps Extension
Weight								
Reps								
Sets								

JOURNAL NOTES

_____

_____

_____

_____

_____

_____

DATE _____   PHASE   1 2 3 4

Did you meet
your goal?

Water (8-ounce glasses)   Limit Alcoholic Beverages
Y N   Y N

Limit Saturated Fat   Limit Refined Carbohydrates

Did you meet
your goal?
Y N   Y N

Fruits   Vegetables   Whole Grains

Did you meet
your goal?
Y N   Y N   Y N

Functional
Exercise Sets   1   2   3

Did you meet
your goal?
Y N   Aerobic Minutes _____
                            Y N

STRENGTH TRAINING   (min. of 3 days/wk)   *(Phase Four only)*

Did you meet your goal? Y   N

	Squat	Lunge	Chest Press	Shoulder Press	Butterfly	Dumbbell Fly	Biceps Curl	Triceps Extension
Weight								
Reps								
Sets								

JOURNAL NOTES

_____

_____

_____

_____

_____

DATE _____   PHASE   1 2 3 4

Did you meet
your goal?   Water (8-ounce glasses)   Limit Alcoholic Beverages
               Y N   Y N

Did you meet   Limit Saturated Fat   Limit Refined Carbohydrates
your goal?   Y N   Y N

Did you meet   Fruits   Vegetables   Whole Grains
your goal?   Y N   Y N   Y N

Did you meet   Functional
your goal?   Exercise Sets 1 2 3   Aerobic Minutes _____
               Y N   Y N

STRENGTH TRAINING   (min. of 3 days/wk)   *(Phase Four only)*

Did you meet your goal? Y N

	Squat	Lunge	Chest Press	Shoulder Press	Butterfly	Dumbbell Fly	Biceps Curl	Triceps Extension
Weight								
Reps								
Sets								

JOURNAL NOTES

_____

_____

_____

_____

_____

_____

DATE _____   PHASE 1 2 3 4

Did you meet
your goal?

Water (8-ounce glasses)   Limit Alcoholic Beverages
Y N   Y N

Limit Saturated Fat   Limit Refined Carbohydrates

Did you meet
your goal?

Y N   Y N

Did you meet
your goal?

Fruits   Vegetables   Whole Grains
Y N   Y N   Y N

Did you meet
your goal?

Functional
Exercise Sets 1 2 3
Y N   Aerobic Minutes _____
                            Y N

STRENGTH TRAINING   (min. of 3 days/wk)   *(Phase Four only)*

Did you meet your goal? Y N

	Squat	Lunge	Chest Press	Shoulder Press	Butterfly	Dumbbell Fly	Biceps Curl	Triceps Extension
Weight								
Reps								
Sets								

JOURNAL NOTES

_____

_____

_____

_____

_____

_____

> *Powerful results in any area of your life*
> *are best accomplished in small increments.*
> *Getting fit is no exception.*

_____

_____

_____

_____

_____

_____

_____

_____

_____

_____

_____

_____

_____

_____

_____

WEEKLY SUMMARY   *Body Weight*_____

	Water (8-ounce Glasses)	Functional Exercises	Aerobic Minutes	Number Alcoholic Beverages	Strength Training Sessions	"Limit 24-7" (All four)	Good Day or Not?
Monday							
Tuesday							
Wednesday							
Thursday							
Friday							
Saturday							
Sunday							

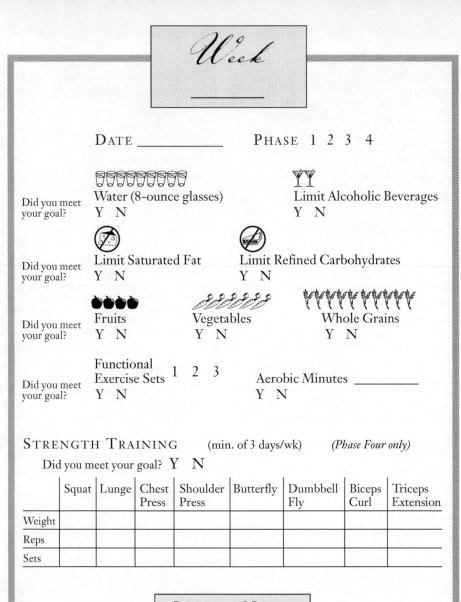

Week

_____

DATE _____   PHASE 1 2 3 4

Did you meet
your goal?   Water (8-ounce glasses)   Limit Alcoholic Beverages
Y N   Y N

Did you meet
your goal?   Limit Saturated Fat   Limit Refined Carbohydrates
Y N   Y N

Did you meet
your goal?   Fruits   Vegetables   Whole Grains
Y N   Y N   Y N

Did you meet
your goal?   Functional
Exercise Sets 1 2 3   Aerobic Minutes _____
Y N   Y N

STRENGTH TRAINING   (min. of 3 days/wk)   *(Phase Four only)*

Did you meet your goal? Y N

	Squat	Lunge	Chest Press	Shoulder Press	Butterfly	Dumbbell Fly	Biceps Curl	Triceps Extension
Weight								
Reps								
Sets								

JOURNAL NOTES

_____

_____

_____

_____

_____

_____

Challenges add meaning to life and represent opportunities for you to grow.

_____

_____

_____

_____

_____

_____

_____

_____

_____

_____

_____

_____

_____

_____

_____

_____

_____

_____

_____

_____

_____

_____

_____

_____

DATE _____   PHASE 1 2 3 4

Did you meet your goal? Water (8-ounce glasses)
Y N

Limit Alcoholic Beverages
Y N

Did you meet your goal? Limit Saturated Fat
Y N

Limit Refined Carbohydrates
Y N

Did you meet your goal? Fruits
Y N

Vegetables
Y N

Whole Grains
Y N

Did you meet your goal? Functional Exercise Sets 1 2 3
Y N

Aerobic Minutes _____
Y N

STRENGTH TRAINING   (min. of 3 days/wk)   *(Phase Four only)*

Did you meet your goal? Y N

	Squat	Lunge	Chest Press	Shoulder Press	Butterfly	Dumbbell Fly	Biceps Curl	Triceps Extension
Weight								
Reps								
Sets								

JOURNAL NOTES

_____

_____

_____

_____

_____

_____

DATE _____   PHASE   1   2   3   4

Did you meet
your goal?
Water (8-ounce glasses)
Y   N

Limit Alcoholic Beverages
Y   N

Did you meet
your goal?
Limit Saturated Fat
Y   N

Limit Refined Carbohydrates
Y   N

Did you meet
your goal?
Fruits
Y   N

Vegetables
Y   N

Whole Grains
Y   N

Did you meet
your goal?
Functional
Exercise Sets   1   2   3
Y   N

Aerobic Minutes _____
Y   N

STRENGTH TRAINING   (min. of 3 days/wk)   *(Phase Four only)*

Did you meet your goal?   Y   N

	Squat	Lunge	Chest Press	Shoulder Press	Butterfly	Dumbbell Fly	Biceps Curl	Triceps Extension
Weight								
Reps								
Sets								

JOURNAL NOTES

_____

_____

_____

_____

_____

_____

DATE _____   PHASE   1   2   3   4

Did you meet
your goal?   Water (8-ounce glasses)   Limit Alcoholic Beverages
                     Y   N   Y   N

Did you meet   Limit Saturated Fat   Limit Refined Carbohydrates
your goal?   Y   N   Y   N

Did you meet   Fruits   Vegetables   Whole Grains
your goal?   Y   N   Y   N   Y   N

Did you meet   Functional
your goal?   Exercise Sets   1   2   3   Aerobic Minutes _____
                     Y   N   Y   N

STRENGTH TRAINING   (min. of 3 days/wk)   *(Phase Four only)*

Did you meet your goal?   Y   N

	Squat	Lunge	Chest Press	Shoulder Press	Butterfly	Dumbbell Fly	Biceps Curl	Triceps Extension
Weight								
Reps								
Sets								

JOURNAL NOTES

_____

_____

_____

_____

_____

_____

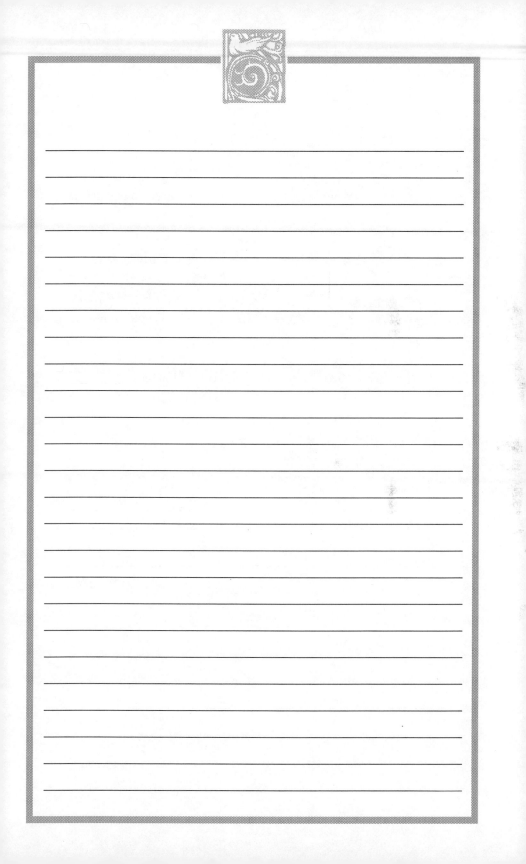

DATE _____   PHASE 1 2 3 4

Did you meet
your goal?
Water (8-ounce glasses)
Y N

Limit Alcoholic Beverages
Y N

Did you meet
your goal?
Limit Saturated Fat
Y N

Limit Refined Carbohydrates
Y N

Did you meet
your goal?
Fruits
Y N

Vegetables
Y N

Whole Grains
Y N

Did you meet
your goal?
Functional
Exercise Sets 1 2 3
Y N

Aerobic Minutes _____
Y N

STRENGTH TRAINING   (min. of 3 days/wk)   *(Phase Four only)*

Did you meet your goal? Y N

	Squat	Lunge	Chest Press	Shoulder Press	Butterfly	Dumbbell Fly	Biceps Curl	Triceps Extension
Weight								
Reps								
Sets								

JOURNAL NOTES

_____

_____

_____

_____

_____

_____

DATE _____   PHASE 1 2 3 4

Did you meet your goal? Water (8-ounce glasses)
Y N

Limit Alcoholic Beverages
Y N

Did you meet your goal? Limit Saturated Fat
Y N

Limit Refined Carbohydrates
Y N

Did you meet your goal? Fruits
Y N

Vegetables
Y N

Whole Grains
Y N

Did you meet your goal? Functional Exercise Sets 1 2 3
Y N

Aerobic Minutes _____
Y N

STRENGTH TRAINING   (min. of 3 days/wk)   *(Phase Four only)*

Did you meet your goal? Y N

	Squat	Lunge	Chest Press	Shoulder Press	Butterfly	Dumbbell Fly	Biceps Curl	Triceps Extension
Weight								
Reps								
Sets								

JOURNAL NOTES

_____

_____

_____

_____

_____

_____

DATE _____   PHASE 1 2 3 4

Did you meet
your goal?

Water (8-ounce glasses)
Y N

Limit Alcoholic Beverages
Y N

Did you meet
your goal?

Limit Saturated Fat
Y N

Limit Refined Carbohydrates
Y N

Did you meet
your goal?

Fruits
Y N

Vegetables
Y N

Whole Grains
Y N

Did you meet
your goal?

Functional
Exercise Sets   1   2   3
Y N

Aerobic Minutes _____
Y N

STRENGTH TRAINING   (min. of 3 days/wk)   *(Phase Four only)*

Did you meet your goal? Y N

	Squat	Lunge	Chest Press	Shoulder Press	Butterfly	Dumbbell Fly	Biceps Curl	Triceps Extension
Weight								
Reps								
Sets								

JOURNAL NOTES

_____

_____

_____

_____

_____

_____

Take the time to acknowledge and praise yourself each day that you stick with your chosen path to your goals, underline especially when your results are slow.

_____

_____

_____

_____

_____

_____

_____

_____

_____

_____

_____

_____

_____

WEEKLY SUMMARY   *Body Weight*_____

	Water (8-ounce Glasses)	Functional Exercises	Aerobic Minutes	Number Alcoholic Beverages	Strength Training Sessions	"Limit 24-7" (All four)	Good Day or Not?
Monday							
Tuesday							
Wednesday							
Thursday							
Friday							
Saturday							
Sunday							

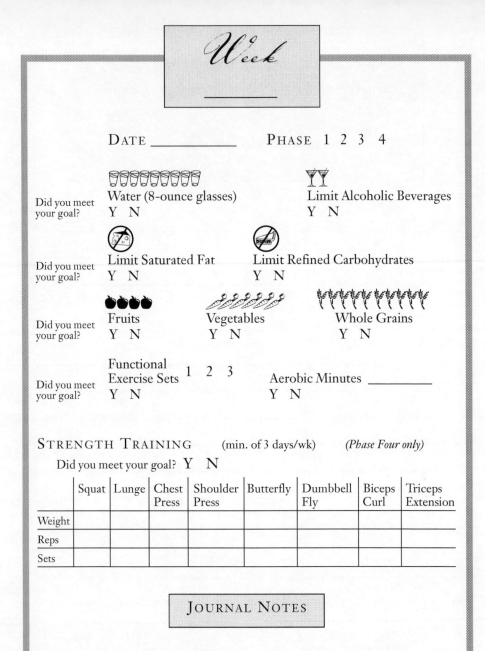

Week

DATE _____   PHASE 1 2 3 4

Did you meet your goal?
Water (8-ounce glasses)
Y N

Limit Alcoholic Beverages
Y N

Did you meet your goal?
Limit Saturated Fat
Y N

Limit Refined Carbohydrates
Y N

Did you meet your goal?
Fruits
Y N

Vegetables
Y N

Whole Grains
Y N

Did you meet your goal?
Functional Exercise Sets   1   2   3
Y N

Aerobic Minutes _____
Y N

STRENGTH TRAINING   (min. of 3 days/wk)   *(Phase Four only)*

Did you meet your goal? Y N

	Squat	Lunge	Chest Press	Shoulder Press	Butterfly	Dumbbell Fly	Biceps Curl	Triceps Extension
Weight								
Reps								
Sets								

JOURNAL NOTES

_____

_____

_____

_____

_____

_____

> *When you do find the courage to risk change*
> *and experience it, even in small doses,*
> *you're in for a powerfully wonderful,*
> *life-changing experience.*

_____
_____
_____
_____
_____
_____
_____
_____
_____
_____
_____
_____
_____
_____
_____
_____
_____
_____
_____
_____
_____
_____
_____
_____
_____
_____

DATE _____   PHASE 1 2 3 4

Did you meet
your goal?
Water (8-ounce glasses)
Y N

Limit Alcoholic Beverages
Y N

Did you meet
your goal?
Limit Saturated Fat
Y N

Limit Refined Carbohydrates
Y N

Did you meet
your goal?
Fruits
Y N

Vegetables
Y N

Whole Grains
Y N

Did you meet
your goal?
Functional
Exercise Sets 1 2 3
Y N

Aerobic Minutes _____
Y N

STRENGTH TRAINING   (min. of 3 days/wk)   *(Phase Four only)*

Did you meet your goal? Y N

	Squat	Lunge	Chest Press	Shoulder Press	Butterfly	Dumbbell Fly	Biceps Curl	Triceps Extension
Weight								
Reps								
Sets								

JOURNAL NOTES

_____

_____

_____

_____

_____

_____

DATE _____   PHASE 1 2 3 4

Did you meet your goal?   Water (8-ounce glasses)   Limit Alcoholic Beverages
Y N   Y N

Did you meet your goal?   Limit Saturated Fat   Limit Refined Carbohydrates
Y N   Y N

Did you meet your goal?   Fruits   Vegetables   Whole Grains
Y N   Y N   Y N

Did you meet your goal?   Functional Exercise Sets 1 2 3   Aerobic Minutes _____
Y N   Y N

STRENGTH TRAINING   (min. of 3 days/wk)   *(Phase Four only)*

Did you meet your goal? Y N

	Squat	Lunge	Chest Press	Shoulder Press	Butterfly	Dumbbell Fly	Biceps Curl	Triceps Extension
Weight								
Reps								
Sets								

JOURNAL NOTES

_____

_____

_____

_____

_____

_____

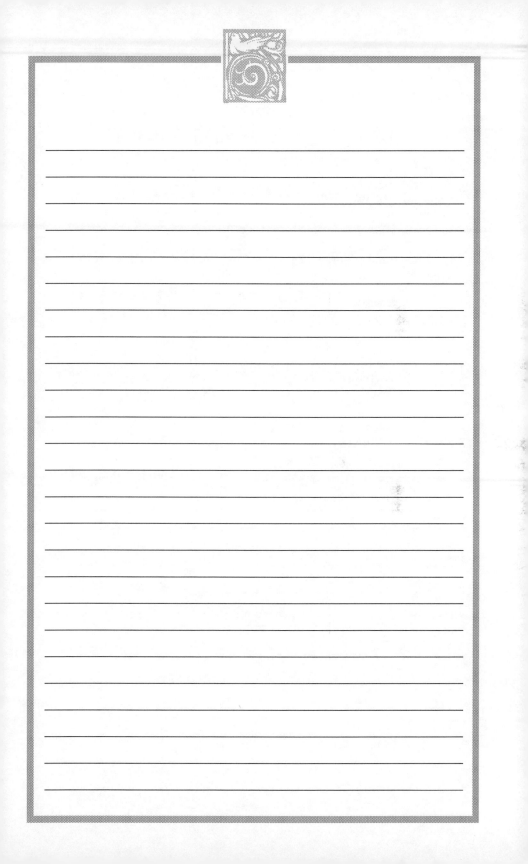

DATE _____   PHASE 1 2 3 4

Did you meet
your goal?

Water (8-ounce glasses)   Limit Alcoholic Beverages
Y N   Y N

Did you meet
your goal?

Limit Saturated Fat   Limit Refined Carbohydrates
Y N   Y N

Did you meet
your goal?

Fruits   Vegetables   Whole Grains
Y N   Y N   Y N

Did you meet
your goal?

Functional
Exercise Sets 1 2 3   Aerobic Minutes _____
Y N   Y N

STRENGTH TRAINING   (min. of 3 days/wk)   *(Phase Four only)*

Did you meet your goal? Y N

	Squat	Lunge	Chest Press	Shoulder Press	Butterfly	Dumbbell Fly	Biceps Curl	Triceps Extension
Weight								
Reps								
Sets								

JOURNAL NOTES

_____

_____

_____

_____

_____

_____

DATE _____ PHASE 1 2 3 4

Did you meet your goal?
Water (8-ounce glasses)
Y N

Limit Alcoholic Beverages
Y N

Did you meet your goal?
Limit Saturated Fat
Y N

Limit Refined Carbohydrates
Y N

Did you meet your goal?
Fruits
Y N

Vegetables
Y N

Whole Grains
Y N

Did you meet your goal?
Functional Exercise Sets 1 2 3
Y N

Aerobic Minutes _____
Y N

STRENGTH TRAINING (min. of 3 days/wk) *(Phase Four only)*

Did you meet your goal? Y N

	Squat	Lunge	Chest Press	Shoulder Press	Butterfly	Dumbbell Fly	Biceps Curl	Triceps Extension
Weight								
Reps								
Sets								

JOURNAL NOTES

_____

_____

_____

_____

_____

_____

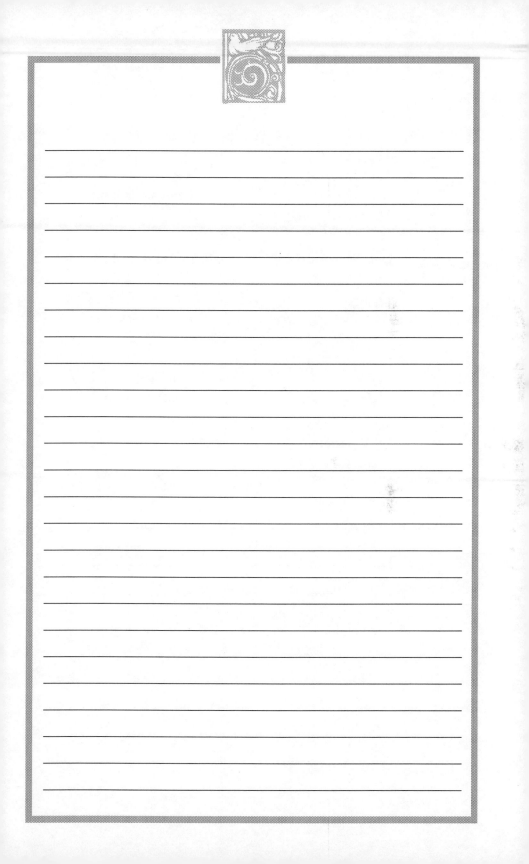

DATE _____   PHASE 1 2 3 4

Did you meet
your goal?
Water (8-ounce glasses)
Y N

Limit Alcoholic Beverages
Y N

Did you meet
your goal?
Limit Saturated Fat
Y N

Limit Refined Carbohydrates
Y N

Did you meet
your goal?
Fruits
Y N

Vegetables
Y N

Whole Grains
Y N

Did you meet
your goal?
Functional
Exercise Sets 1 2 3
Y N

Aerobic Minutes _____
Y N

STRENGTH TRAINING   (min. of 3 days/wk)   *(Phase Four only)*

Did you meet your goal? Y N

	Squat	Lunge	Chest Press	Shoulder Press	Butterfly	Dumbbell Fly	Biceps Curl	Triceps Extension
Weight								
Reps								
Sets								

JOURNAL NOTES

_____

_____

_____

_____

_____

_____

DATE _____ PHASE 1 2 3 4

Did you meet
your goal?

Water (8-ounce glasses)
Y N

Limit Alcoholic Beverages
Y N

Did you meet
your goal?

Limit Saturated Fat
Y N

Limit Refined Carbohydrates
Y N

Did you meet
your goal?

Fruits
Y N

Vegetables
Y N

Whole Grains
Y N

Did you meet
your goal?

Functional
Exercise Sets   1   2   3
Y N

Aerobic Minutes _____
Y N

STRENGTH TRAINING   (min. of 3 days/wk)   *(Phase Four only)*

Did you meet your goal? Y N

	Squat	Lunge	Chest Press	Shoulder Press	Butterfly	Dumbbell Fly	Biceps Curl	Triceps Extension
Weight								
Reps								
Sets								

JOURNAL NOTES

_____

_____

_____

_____

_____

_____

Results come from focusing on knowing
what you want, renewing your commitment to
yourself each day, and improving the things
that you can one small step at a time.

_____

_____

_____

_____

_____

_____

_____

_____

_____

_____

_____

_____

_____

WEEKLY SUMMARY   *Body Weight*_____

	Water (8-ounce Glasses)	Functional Exercises	Aerobic Minutes	Number Alcoholic Beverages	Strength Training Sessions	"Limit 24-7" (All four)	Good Day or Not?
Monday							
Tuesday							
Wednesday							
Thursday							
Friday							
Saturday							
Sunday							

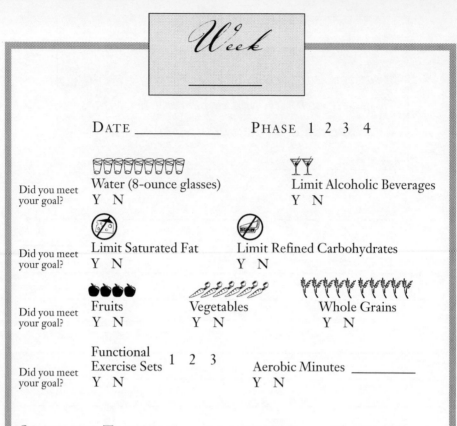

$$\mathcal{W}eek$$

_____

DATE _____ PHASE 1 2 3 4

Did you meet
your goal?
Water (8-ounce glasses)
Y N

Limit Alcoholic Beverages
Y N

Did you meet
your goal?
Limit Saturated Fat
Y N

Limit Refined Carbohydrates
Y N

Did you meet
your goal?
Fruits
Y N

Vegetables
Y N

Whole Grains
Y N

Did you meet
your goal?
Functional
Exercise Sets 1 2 3
Y N

Aerobic Minutes _____
Y N

STRENGTH TRAINING (min. of 3 days/wk) _(Phase Four only)_

Did you meet your goal? Y N

	Squat	Lunge	Chest Press	Shoulder Press	Butterfly	Dumbbell Fly	Biceps Curl	Triceps Extension
Weight								
Reps								
Sets								

JOURNAL NOTES

_____

_____

_____

_____

_____

_____

> *Caring about yourself and doing good things for yourself is not only your right, it's your responsibility.*

_____
_____
_____
_____
_____
_____
_____
_____
_____
_____
_____
_____
_____
_____
_____
_____
_____
_____
_____
_____
_____
_____
_____
_____

DATE _____   PHASE 1 2 3 4

Did you meet
your goal?   Water (8-ounce glasses)   Limit Alcoholic Beverages
              Y N   Y N

Did you meet
your goal?   Limit Saturated Fat   Limit Refined Carbohydrates
              Y N   Y N

Did you meet
your goal?   Fruits   Vegetables   Whole Grains
              Y N   Y N   Y N

Did you meet   Functional
your goal?   Exercise Sets 1 2 3
                Y N   Aerobic Minutes _____
                                        Y N

STRENGTH TRAINING   (min. of 3 days/wk)   *(Phase Four only)*

Did you meet your goal? Y N

	Squat	Lunge	Chest Press	Shoulder Press	Butterfly	Dumbbell Fly	Biceps Curl	Triceps Extension
Weight								
Reps								
Sets								

JOURNAL NOTES

_____

_____

_____

_____

_____

_____

DATE _____   PHASE 1 2 3 4

Did you meet your goal?
Water (8-ounce glasses)
Y N

Limit Alcoholic Beverages
Y N

Did you meet your goal?
Limit Saturated Fat
Y N

Limit Refined Carbohydrates
Y N

Did you meet your goal?
Fruits
Y N

Vegetables
Y N

Whole Grains
Y N

Did you meet your goal?
Functional Exercise Sets 1 2 3
Y N

Aerobic Minutes _____
Y N

STRENGTH TRAINING   (min. of 3 days/wk)   *(Phase Four only)*

Did you meet your goal? Y N

	Squat	Lunge	Chest Press	Shoulder Press	Butterfly	Dumbbell Fly	Biceps Curl	Triceps Extension
Weight								
Reps								
Sets								

JOURNAL NOTES

_____

_____

_____

_____

_____

_____

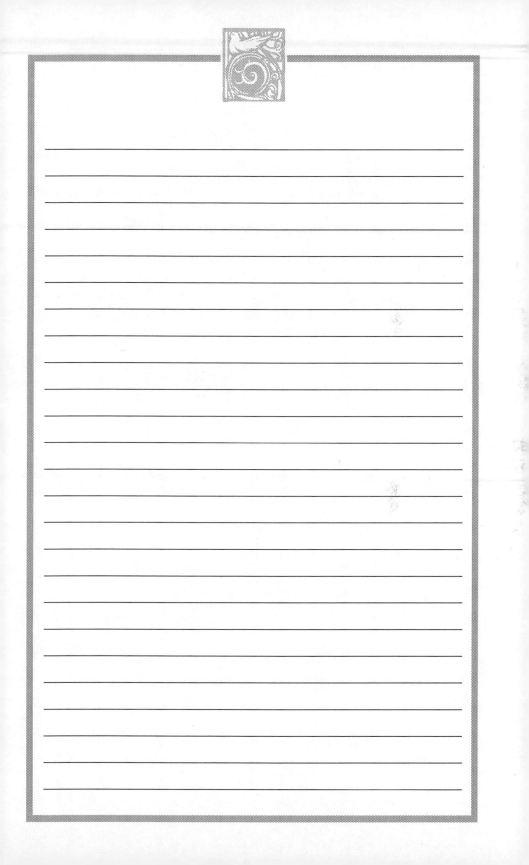

DATE _____   PHASE 1 2 3 4

Did you meet your goal?   Water (8-ounce glasses)   Limit Alcoholic Beverages
                          Y N   Y N

Did you meet your goal?   Limit Saturated Fat   Limit Refined Carbohydrates
                          Y N   Y N

Did you meet your goal?   Fruits   Vegetables   Whole Grains
                          Y N   Y N   Y N

Did you meet your goal?   Functional
                          Exercise Sets 1 2 3   Aerobic Minutes _____
                          Y N   Y N

STRENGTH TRAINING   (min. of 3 days/wk)   *(Phase Four only)*

Did you meet your goal? Y N

	Squat	Lunge	Chest Press	Shoulder Press	Butterfly	Dumbbell Fly	Biceps Curl	Triceps Extension
Weight								
Reps								
Sets								

JOURNAL NOTES

_____

_____

_____

_____

_____

_____

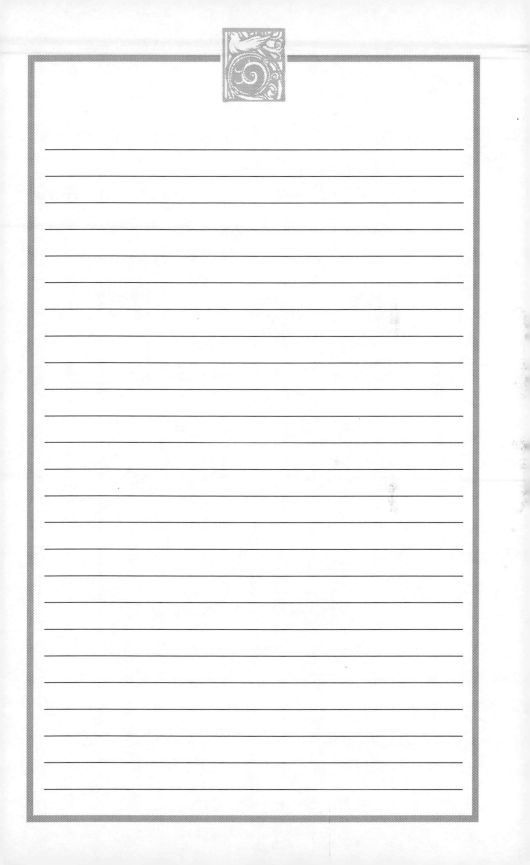

DATE _____   PHASE 1 2 3 4

Did you meet
your goal?
Water (8-ounce glasses)   Limit Alcoholic Beverages
Y N   Y N

Did you meet
your goal?
Limit Saturated Fat   Limit Refined Carbohydrates
Y N   Y N

Did you meet
your goal?
Fruits   Vegetables   Whole Grains
Y N   Y N   Y N

Did you meet
your goal?
Functional
Exercise Sets 1 2 3
Y N   Aerobic Minutes _____
                        Y N

STRENGTH TRAINING   (min. of 3 days/wk)   *(Phase Four only)*
    Did you meet your goal? Y N

	Squat	Lunge	Chest Press	Shoulder Press	Butterfly	Dumbbell Fly	Biceps Curl	Triceps Extension
Weight								
Reps								
Sets								

JOURNAL NOTES

_____

_____

_____

_____

_____

_____

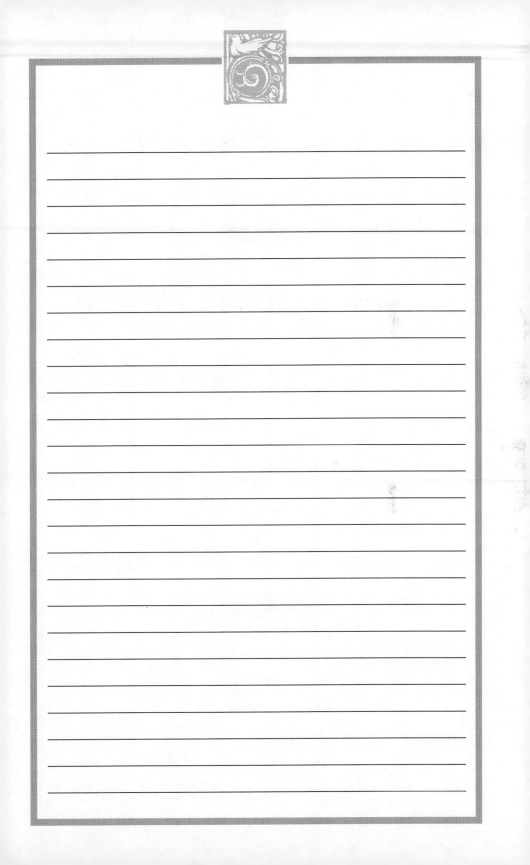

DATE _____   PHASE 1 2 3 4

Did you meet your goal?   🥛🥛🥛🥛🥛🥛🥛🥛 Water (8-ounce glasses)
Y N

🍸🍸 Limit Alcoholic Beverages
Y N

Did you meet your goal?   🚫 Limit Saturated Fat
Y N

🚫 Limit Refined Carbohydrates
Y N

Did you meet your goal?   🍎🍎🍎🍎 Fruits
Y N

🥕🥕🥕🥕🥕 Vegetables
Y N

🌾🌾🌾🌾🌾🌾🌾🌾🌾🌾🌾 Whole Grains
Y N

Did you meet your goal?   Functional Exercise Sets 1 2 3
Y N

Aerobic Minutes _____
Y N

STRENGTH TRAINING   (min. of 3 days/wk)   *(Phase Four only)*
Did you meet your goal? Y N

	Squat	Lunge	Chest Press	Shoulder Press	Butterfly	Dumbbell Fly	Biceps Curl	Triceps Extension
Weight								
Reps								
Sets								

JOURNAL NOTES

_____

_____

_____

_____

_____

_____

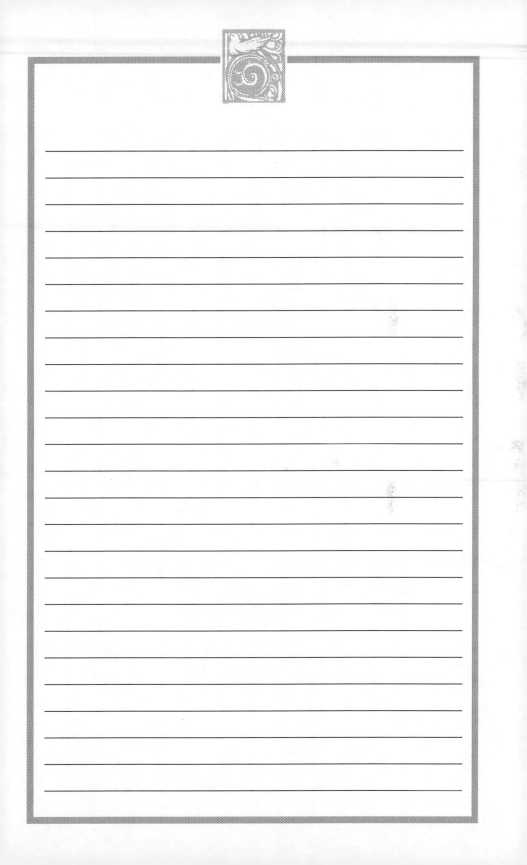

DATE _____   PHASE 1 2 3 4

Did you meet your goal?   Water (8-ounce glasses)   Limit Alcoholic Beverages
                          Y N   Y N

Did you meet your goal?   Limit Saturated Fat   Limit Refined Carbohydrates
                          Y N   Y N

Did you meet your goal?   Fruits   Vegetables   Whole Grains
                          Y N   Y N   Y N

Did you meet your goal?   Functional Exercise Sets 1 2 3   Aerobic Minutes _____
                          Y N   Y N

STRENGTH TRAINING   (min. of 3 days/wk)   *(Phase Four only)*

Did you meet your goal? Y N

	Squat	Lunge	Chest Press	Shoulder Press	Butterfly	Dumbbell Fly	Biceps Curl	Triceps Extension
Weight								
Reps								
Sets								

JOURNAL NOTES

_____

_____

_____

_____

_____

_____

As long as you are patient and believe you are doing the best thing for yourself and that you deserve the results you desire, those results will happen.

_____
_____
_____
_____
_____
_____
_____
_____
_____
_____
_____
_____
_____
_____

WEEKLY SUMMARY   *Body Weight*_____

	Water (8-ounce Glasses)	Functional Exercises	Aerobic Minutes	Number Alcoholic Beverages	Strength Training Sessions	"Limit 24-7" (All four)	Good Day or Not?
Monday							
Tuesday							
Wednesday							
Thursday							
Friday							
Saturday							
Sunday							

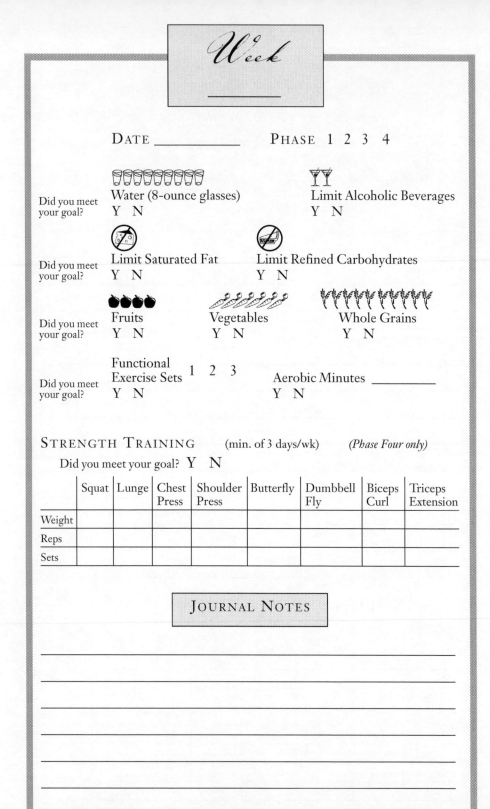

Week
_____

DATE _____   PHASE 1 2 3 4

Did you meet your goal? Water (8-ounce glasses)   Limit Alcoholic Beverages
Y N   Y N

Did you meet your goal? Limit Saturated Fat   Limit Refined Carbohydrates
Y N   Y N

Did you meet your goal? Fruits   Vegetables   Whole Grains
Y N   Y N   Y N

Did you meet your goal? Functional Exercise Sets 1 2 3   Aerobic Minutes _____
Y N   Y N

STRENGTH TRAINING   (min. of 3 days/wk)   *(Phase Four only)*

Did you meet your goal? Y N

	Squat	Lunge	Chest Press	Shoulder Press	Butterfly	Dumbbell Fly	Biceps Curl	Triceps Extension
Weight								
Reps								
Sets								

JOURNAL NOTES

_____

_____

_____

_____

_____

_____

Living the best possible life is everyone's dream.

DATE _____   PHASE   1 2 3 4

Did you meet
your goal?
Water (8-ounce glasses)
Y N

Limit Alcoholic Beverages
Y N

Did you meet
your goal?
Limit Saturated Fat
Y N

Limit Refined Carbohydrates
Y N

Did you meet
your goal?
Fruits
Y N

Vegetables
Y N

Whole Grains
Y N

Did you meet
your goal?
Functional
Exercise Sets   1   2   3
Y N

Aerobic Minutes _____
Y N

STRENGTH TRAINING   (min. of 3 days/wk)   *(Phase Four only)*

Did you meet your goal? Y N

	Squat	Lunge	Chest Press	Shoulder Press	Butterfly	Dumbbell Fly	Biceps Curl	Triceps Extension
Weight								
Reps								
Sets								

JOURNAL NOTES

_____

_____

_____

_____

_____

_____

DATE _____   PHASE 1 2 3 4

Did you meet   Water (8-ounce glasses)   Limit Alcoholic Beverages
your goal?   Y N   Y N

Did you meet   Limit Saturated Fat   Limit Refined Carbohydrates
your goal?   Y N   Y N

Did you meet   Fruits   Vegetables   Whole Grains
your goal?   Y N   Y N   Y N

Did you meet   Functional
your goal?   Exercise Sets 1 2 3   Aerobic Minutes _____
                  Y N   Y N

STRENGTH TRAINING   (min. of 3 days/wk)   *(Phase Four only)*

Did you meet your goal? Y N

	Squat	Lunge	Chest Press	Shoulder Press	Butterfly	Dumbbell Fly	Biceps Curl	Triceps Extension
Weight								
Reps								
Sets								

JOURNAL NOTES

_____

_____

_____

_____

_____

_____

DATE _____   PHASE 1 2 3 4

Did you meet
your goal?   Water (8-ounce glasses)   Limit Alcoholic Beverages
                    Y N   Y N

Did you meet   Limit Saturated Fat   Limit Refined Carbohydrates
your goal?   Y N   Y N

Did you meet   Fruits   Vegetables   Whole Grains
your goal?   Y N   Y N   Y N

Did you meet   Functional
your goal?   Exercise Sets   1   2   3   Aerobic Minutes _____
                    Y N   Y N

STRENGTH TRAINING   (min. of 3 days/wk)   *(Phase Four only)*

Did you meet your goal? Y   N

	Squat	Lunge	Chest Press	Shoulder Press	Butterfly	Dumbbell Fly	Biceps Curl	Triceps Extension
Weight								
Reps								
Sets								

JOURNAL NOTES

_____

_____

_____

_____

_____

_____

DATE _____   PHASE 1 2 3 4

Did you meet
your goal?   Water (8-ounce glasses)   Limit Alcoholic Beverages
                  Y N   Y N

Did you meet
your goal?   Limit Saturated Fat   Limit Refined Carbohydrates
                  Y N   Y N

Did you meet   Fruits   Vegetables   Whole Grains
your goal?   Y N   Y N   Y N

Did you meet   Functional
your goal?   Exercise Sets 1 2 3   Aerobic Minutes _____
                  Y N   Y N

STRENGTH TRAINING   (min. of 3 days/wk)   *(Phase Four only)*

Did you meet your goal? Y N

	Squat	Lunge	Chest Press	Shoulder Press	Butterfly	Dumbbell Fly	Biceps Curl	Triceps Extension
Weight								
Reps								
Sets								

JOURNAL NOTES

_____

_____

_____

_____

_____

_____

DATE _____   PHASE 1 2 3 4

Did you meet
your goal?   Water (8-ounce glasses)   Limit Alcoholic Beverages
                  Y N   Y N

Did you meet   Limit Saturated Fat   Limit Refined Carbohydrates
your goal?   Y N   Y N

Did you meet   Fruits   Vegetables   Whole Grains
your goal?   Y N   Y N   Y N

Did you meet   Functional
your goal?   Exercise Sets 1 2 3   Aerobic Minutes _____
                  Y N   Y N

STRENGTH TRAINING   (min. of 3 days/wk)   *(Phase Four only)*

Did you meet your goal? Y N

	Squat	Lunge	Chest Press	Shoulder Press	Butterfly	Dumbbell Fly	Biceps Curl	Triceps Extension
Weight								
Reps								
Sets								

JOURNAL NOTES

_____

_____

_____

_____

_____

_____

DATE _____   PHASE   1   2   3   4

Did you meet
your goal?
Water (8-ounce glasses)
Y   N

Limit Alcoholic Beverages
Y   N

Did you meet
your goal?
Limit Saturated Fat
Y   N

Limit Refined Carbohydrates
Y   N

Did you meet
your goal?
Fruits
Y   N

Vegetables
Y   N

Whole Grains
Y   N

Did you meet
your goal?
Functional
Exercise Sets   1   2   3
Y   N

Aerobic Minutes _____
Y   N

STRENGTH TRAINING   (min. of 3 days/wk)   *(Phase Four only)*

Did you meet your goal?   Y   N

	Squat	Lunge	Chest Press	Shoulder Press	Butterfly	Dumbbell Fly	Biceps Curl	Triceps Extension
Weight								
Reps								
Sets								

JOURNAL NOTES

_____

_____

_____

_____

_____

_____

_____
_____
_____
_____
_____
_____
_____
_____
_____
_____
_____
_____
_____
_____
_____
_____
_____
_____
_____

WEEKLY SUMMARY   *Body Weight*_____

	Water (8-ounce Glasses)	Functional Exercises	Aerobic Minutes	Number Alcoholic Beverages	Strength Training Sessions	"Limit 24-7" (All four)	Good Day or Not?
Monday							
Tuesday							
Wednesday							
Thursday							
Friday							
Saturday							
Sunday							

$$\mathscr{Week}$$

_____

DATE _____   PHASE 1 2 3 4

Did you meet your goal?   Water (8-ounce glasses)   Limit Alcoholic Beverages
Y N   Y N

Did you meet your goal?   Limit Saturated Fat   Limit Refined Carbohydrates
Y N   Y N

Did you meet your goal?   Fruits   Vegetables   Whole Grains
Y N   Y N   Y N

Did you meet your goal?   Functional
Exercise Sets 1 2 3   Aerobic Minutes _____
Y N   Y N

STRENGTH TRAINING   (min. of 3 days/wk)   _(Phase Four only)_
Did you meet your goal? Y N

	Squat	Lunge	Chest Press	Shoulder Press	Butterfly	Dumbbell Fly	Biceps Curl	Triceps Extension
Weight								
Reps								
Sets								

JOURNAL NOTES

_____

_____

_____

_____

_____

_____

> *The entire premise behind training is to challenge your body and have it respond by getting stronger. Don't challenge it and risk having little or no change take place.*

_____

_____

_____

_____

_____

_____

_____

_____

_____

_____

_____

_____

_____

_____

_____

_____

_____

_____

_____

_____

_____

_____

_____

_____

DATE _____   PHASE 1 2 3 4

Did you meet
your goal?

Water (8-ounce glasses)
Y N

Limit Alcoholic Beverages
Y N

Did you meet
your goal?

Limit Saturated Fat
Y N

Limit Refined Carbohydrates
Y N

Did you meet
your goal?

Fruits
Y N

Vegetables
Y N

Whole Grains
Y N

Did you meet
your goal?

Functional
Exercise Sets 1   2   3
Y N

Aerobic Minutes _____
Y N

STRENGTH TRAINING   (min. of 3 days/wk)   *(Phase Four only)*

Did you meet your goal? Y N

	Squat	Lunge	Chest Press	Shoulder Press	Butterfly	Dumbbell Fly	Biceps Curl	Triceps Extension
Weight								
Reps								
Sets								

JOURNAL NOTES

_____

_____

_____

_____

_____

_____

DATE _____ PHASE 1 2 3 4

Did you meet your goal?   Water (8-ounce glasses)
Y N

Limit Alcoholic Beverages
Y N

Did you meet your goal?   Limit Saturated Fat
Y N

Limit Refined Carbohydrates
Y N

Did you meet your goal?   Fruits
Y N

Vegetables
Y N

Whole Grains
Y N

Did you meet your goal?   Functional Exercise Sets 1 2 3
Y N

Aerobic Minutes _____
Y N

STRENGTH TRAINING   (min. of 3 days/wk)   *(Phase Four only)*

Did you meet your goal? Y N

	Squat	Lunge	Chest Press	Shoulder Press	Butterfly	Dumbbell Fly	Biceps Curl	Triceps Extension
Weight								
Reps								
Sets								

JOURNAL NOTES

_____

_____

_____

_____

_____

_____

DATE _____   PHASE 1 2 3 4

Did you meet your goal? Water (8-ounce glasses)
Y N

Limit Alcoholic Beverages
Y N

Did you meet your goal? Limit Saturated Fat
Y N

Limit Refined Carbohydrates
Y N

Did you meet your goal? Fruits   Vegetables   Whole Grains
Y N   Y N   Y N

Did you meet your goal? Functional Exercise Sets 1 2 3

Aerobic Minutes _____
Y N

STRENGTH TRAINING   (min. of 3 days/wk)   *(Phase Four only)*

Did you meet your goal? Y N

	Squat	Lunge	Chest Press	Shoulder Press	Butterfly	Dumbbell Fly	Biceps Curl	Triceps Extension
Weight								
Reps								
Sets								

JOURNAL NOTES

_____

_____

_____

_____

_____

_____

DATE _____   PHASE   1 2 3   4

Did you meet
your goal?
Water (8-ounce glasses)   Limit Alcoholic Beverages
Y N   Y N

Did you meet
your goal?
Limit Saturated Fat   Limit Refined Carbohydrates
Y N   Y N

Did you meet
your goal?
Fruits   Vegetables   Whole Grains
Y N   Y N   Y N

Did you meet
your goal?
Functional
Exercise Sets   1   2   3
Y N   Aerobic Minutes _____
                        Y N

STRENGTH TRAINING   (min. of 3 days/wk)   *(Phase Four only)*

Did you meet your goal? Y N

	Squat	Lunge	Chest Press	Shoulder Press	Butterfly	Dumbbell Fly	Biceps Curl	Triceps Extension
Weight								
Reps								
Sets								

JOURNAL NOTES

_____

_____

_____

_____

_____

_____

DATE _____ PHASE 1 2 3 4

Did you meet your goal? Water (8-ounce glasses)
Y N

Limit Alcoholic Beverages
Y N

Did you meet your goal? Limit Saturated Fat
Y N

Limit Refined Carbohydrates
Y N

Did you meet your goal? Fruits
Y N

Vegetables
Y N

Whole Grains
Y N

Did you meet your goal? Functional Exercise Sets 1 2 3
Y N

Aerobic Minutes _____
Y N

STRENGTH TRAINING (min. of 3 days/wk) *(Phase Four only)*

Did you meet your goal? Y N

	Squat	Lunge	Chest Press	Shoulder Press	Butterfly	Dumbbell Fly	Biceps Curl	Triceps Extension
Weight								
Reps								
Sets								

JOURNAL NOTES

_____

_____

_____

_____

_____

_____

DATE _____   PHASE   1   2   3   4

Did you meet
your goal?
Water (8-ounce glasses)
Y   N

Limit Alcoholic Beverages
Y   N

Did you meet
your goal?
Limit Saturated Fat
Y   N

Limit Refined Carbohydrates
Y   N

Did you meet
your goal?
Fruits
Y   N

Vegetables
Y   N

Whole Grains
Y   N

Did you meet
your goal?
Functional
Exercise Sets   1   2   3
Y   N

Aerobic Minutes _____
Y   N

STRENGTH TRAINING   (min. of 3 days/wk)   *(Phase Four only)*

Did you meet your goal?   Y   N

	Squat	Lunge	Chest Press	Shoulder Press	Butterfly	Dumbbell Fly	Biceps Curl	Triceps Extension
Weight								
Reps								
Sets								

JOURNAL NOTES

_____

_____

_____

_____

_____

_____

We need to remember that we create ourselves by the choices we make. And while each of us is blessed with individual strengths and weaknesses, what we create with that which we have is what is ultimately meaningful.

_____
_____
_____
_____
_____
_____
_____
_____
_____
_____
_____
_____
_____
_____
_____

WEEKLY SUMMARY   *Body Weight*_____

	Water (8-ounce Glasses)	Functional Exercises	Aerobic Minutes	Number Alcoholic Beverages	Strength Training Sessions	"Limit 24-7" (All four)	Good Day or Not?
Monday							
Tuesday							
Wednesday							
Thursday							
Friday							
Saturday							
Sunday							

JOURNAL NOTES

JOURNAL NOTES

> *Eating should be enjoyed.*
> *It must also become conscious.*

JOURNAL NOTES

JOURNAL NOTES

*Always remember that your
best investment is in yourself.*

> *At the moment that you're most tempted to emotionally eat, your true self is crying out for you to change some aspect of your life.*

_____

_____

_____

_____

_____

_____

_____

_____

_____

_____

_____

_____

_____

_____

_____

_____

_____

_____

_____

_____

_____

_____

JOURNAL NOTES

Caring for yourself is a daily process.

_____
_____
_____
_____
_____
_____
_____
_____
_____
_____
_____
_____
_____
_____
_____
_____
_____
_____
_____
_____
_____
_____
_____

JOURNAL NOTES

JOURNAL NOTES

JOURNAL NOTES

> *Each day of your life you wake up and make the conscious or unconscious choice to either elevate yourself, stay as you are, or slide backwards—in every aspect of your life.*

_____
_____
_____
_____
_____
_____
_____
_____
_____
_____

GENERAL HEALTH INFORMATION

Record your progress below:

Weight_____

Blood Pressure _____Systolic _____Diastolic

Total Cholesterol_____

LDL_____   HDL_____

Blood Glucose_____

Measurements *(optional)*

Chest_____ Waist_____ Hips_____

Don't forget to log on to getwiththeprogram.org
and enjoy your free trial membership today!